Alexander
TECHNIQUE

Richard Craze

TEACH YOURSELF BOOKS

Cover photograph © Bubbles, Jonathan Turner
Line drawings by Su Eaton

Long-renowned as the authoritative source for self-guided learning – with more than 30 million copies sold worldwide – the *Teach Yourself* series includes over 200 titles in the fields of languages, crafts, hobbies, sports, and other leisure activities.

Library of Congress Catalog Number: 95-7130 5

First published in UK 1996 by Hodder Headline Plc, 338 Euston Road, London NW1 3BH

Catalogue entry for this title is available from the British Library.

First published in US 1992 by NTC Publishing Group, 4255 West Touhy Avenue, Lincolnwood (Chicago), Illinois 60646 – 1975 U.S.A.

The 'Teach Yourself' name and logo are registered trade marks of Hodder & Stoughton Ltd in the UK.

Typeset by Transet Limited, Coventry, Warwickshire.
Printed in Great Britain by Cox & Wyman Ltd, Reading, Berkshire.

Impression number	10 9 8 7 6 5 4
Year	1999 1998 1997

This book is dedicated to my mother, Jeanne,
who never once told me
to sit up straight

ACKNOWLEDGEMENTS

The author would like to thank the following people who have helped in the preparation of this book: Richard Brennan, Susan Mears, Ronnie Sway, Doctor Edward Featherstone, Sue Hart, Ros Jay and STAT

CONTENTS

INTRODUCTION

The right thing to do will probably be the last thing we will do, left to ourselves, because it would be the last thing we should think would be the right thing to do.

F M Alexander

What is the Alexander Technique?

As an estimated one million people are off work with backache each week in the UK alone we must be doing something wrong. Doctors usually prescribe painkillers, osteopaths can sometimes correct the problem but often only temporarily, and surgeons can operate. What is needed is a simple but effective method of re-education: unlearning what it is that we are doing wrong in the first place. The Alexander Technique is exactly that. First developed in the early part of this century it has taken its place as a major new process of body care. It has, up until now, usually been practised by 'teachers' who correct the problems and give advice.

Teach Yourself Alexander Technique is a practical guide to learning the Alexander Technique so that you can practise it for yourself; a practical, simple but effective guide; a 'teach-yourself' instruction manual.

It is likely that most people will have heard of the Alexander Technique but probably will not have had a lesson from a qualified teacher. So, although this is a teach-yourself book, it also explains what happens in a lesson. It is primarily written, however, for the consumer; the 'end-user'. Some of the complicated language or jargon of the Alexander Technique has been simplified so that you won't be

— 1 —

made to feel that you are reading a text book and you should, therefore, be able to understand the information more easily.

This book takes you through a series of practical exercises and procedures that you can learn to do at home for yourself. It also explores the added benefits, emotional and mental, of what is essentially a physical approach to good health.

Why Alexander?

We will start with a history of the Technique which must include a brief history of the man who discovered it in the latter part of the last century, Frederick Matthias Alexander.

Alexander was a Tasmanian actor who suffered from a recurring problem of voice loss when he was performing his one-man theatrical recitations of Shakespearean speeches. How he found a cure and went on to develop the Technique is told in Chapter 1.

To understand the principles behind the Alexander Technique it is quite important to know how and why Alexander developed them in the way that he did. Reading about his own personal journey of discovery leads us to a realisation about the Technique itself – what he did, we can also do.

Who can learn it?

There is a nothing difficult or extreme about learning the Alexander Technique. It is a safe and effective form of moving our bodies in the way that they were designed to move. It can be taught to children and adults of all ages and physical conditions. If you are in any doubt about your ability to practise the Technique, however, it would be advisable to check with your doctor or a qualified teacher.

Above all, do not overdo any of the exercises included in this book – take your time, and exercise caution about how and where you practise.

What it isn't

The Alexander Technique is not a therapy, philosophy or creed so you won't be asked to change your diet, lifestyle or the way you dress. Nor will you be asked to 'believe' anything. The Technique works on a fairly simple principle – try it and if it works for you, do it.

We'll have a look at the sort of people who learn it and what they use it for, and why you may want to learn it for yourself. This might include treatment for a specific problem like backache, or to help improve your performance in a special area like dancing or athletics, or just from a general interest point of view – you've heard about it and wondered what it was.

Putting it into practice

We will work through some practical exercises as well as looking at the principles behind the Technique. We will also explore how we can put the Technique into practice in our everyday life – there's no point learning something if we can't benefit from it in a real and practical way. Putting it into practice can be as simple as taking the tension out of sitting down and standing up – or we can use it in complicated applications like learning Tai Ch'i or playing the violin.

Learning the Technique merely requires a certain desire to practise the simple exercises combined with an open mind. If we already have concepts of what the Technique is and isn't, it will be harder for us to let go of our expectations and allow our bodies to move naturally. If we think we *know* what is *right* and what is *wrong*, it will be so much harder for us to learn what is *aligned* and *misaligned* or what is *working well* or *not working well*.

How does it work?

We will also have to look at how the human body works but in a fairly basic way – this isn't going to be a biology lesson. It's just that to understand what we're doing wrong we have to know how it's supposed to work in the way it was designed to work.

Throughout the book we will also look at some practical applications. If there is something you do that is special, like playing the oboe or underwater hang-gliding, that has not been included, don't worry. Once the principles are learnt it doesn't take much to apply them to your own particular application – there will be plenty of tips and advice on how to adapt and apply the Technique.

At the back of the book you'll find some useful information such as the address of the Society of Teachers of the Alexander Technique, as well as information on training, where to get books, how to become an Associate Member and how to find out about classes and workshops.

What's the technique of the Alexander Technique?

And just to clear up a popular misconception, the Alexander Technique isn't a *technique* in the strict sense of the word. It is simply a way of learning to move our bodies in the way that they were designed to be moved. The way we are brought up combined with the stresses and strains of modern living set us in ways of moving that cause us excess tension and misalignment. The Alexander Technique helps us to *unlearn* those habits and regain the supple poise and grace we had when we were young. Once our physical structure is free from tension and aches we automatically adopt a more positive outlook on life and an increase in our emotional well-being; our mental powers improve and we benefit from an all round improvement in the quality of our lives.

Additional benefits

We might set out to learn the Technique to correct a niggling back problem and find ourselves fitter, more supple, happier and more relaxed than we've been in years. We may learn the Technique out of curiosity and find ourselves more active, sleeping better, eating better and suffering from fewer minor ailments. We could even learn the Technique, as many do, to help improve our balance and co-ordination when we are playing a musical instrument, such as the bagpipes, only to find we have improved our breathing, lowered our blood pressure and taken on a new zest and enthusiasm for living. Whatever our reasons for wanting to learn the Technique it can only be beneficial – moving with a natural grace and poise uses less energy, creates less tension and gives us more time to enjoy our lives.

1

A HISTORY OF
THE ALEXANDER
TECHNIQUE

*If people go on believing that they 'know' then it is impossible to
eradicate anything – it becomes impossible to teach them.*

F M Alexander

To understand the Alexander Technique fully it is essential to know
how and why it came about. You may be tempted to skip this chapter
but I would seriously recommend that you don't. Without knowing
who Frederick Matthias Alexander was and how he developed his
Technique you could miss a lot of vital clues as to how it works.

Most books that concern therapies of one sort or another include case
histories, but for the Alexander Technique the best case history is the
man himself.

—— Alexander's early history ——

Alexander was born into a poor family in Wynyard, Tasmania in
1869. He was the eldest of eight children and grew up on a remote
farm in north-west Tasmania. As a child he was weak and sickly, and
suffered from continual breathing problems. Today he may well have
been diagnosed as asthmatic. At times he was too ill to attend school
and was kept at home where he managed to learn whatever he could.
Naturally being at home a lot led to him growing up isolated from
other children. Right from an early age he was individualistic and
unorthodox. He was at that time labelled as precocious.

From the age of about nine his health began to improve although he continued to stay at home. He began to learn how to manage horses, which his family bred, exercising them and training them. The passion for horses stayed with him throughout his life. He also began to show an interest in the theatre – it seemed a natural path for someone as confident and outgoing as Alexander to follow. Remember it was the 1870s, there was no television, not even radio, and he lived on a farm a long way away from the nearest neighbours, with seven younger brothers and sisters. What could be more natural than for him to become the entertainer for their benefit? Alexander discovered Shakespeare around this time and began to learn how to recite his favourite speeches. He set his heart on a life as an actor but in 1885, when he was still only sixteen, the family suffered a series of disastrous financial setbacks and Alexander had no choice but to look around for a regular job.

A young man in Melbourne

Alexander had to take whatever was offered and found himself in the mining town of Mount Bischoff – as a clerk in a tin mine. Somehow he managed to stick at it, sending money home regularly, until three years later when he had managed to save enough to get himself to Melbourne. By now the family's fortunes had revived somewhat and Alexander was able to use his savings to rent board and lodgings in the city and to pay for acting lessons. He also discovered a new passion for music.

He was nineteen years old and living in a big city for the first time. He entered into the spirit of his new life completely. He went to the theatre as often as possible, mixed with other actors, visited art galleries, attended concerts, and even managed to organise his own amateur dramatic company.

Casual work

These were exciting times for the young actor. When he ran short of money he took casual jobs as and when he could find them – as a bookkeeper and a clerk, a store assistant and a tea-taster. He never managed to keep any job for very long for three reasons. First, he despised what he called 'trade'; second, he suffered from a short fuse and a fairly violent temper; and third, he couldn't be bothered to dedicate himself to any job for the simple reason that he knew he was going to be an actor – and a good one.

During his early twenties he had established himself as a fine young actor with a considerable reputation. He developed a one-man show that was a mixture of dramatic and humorous recitals, but his speciality was still his Shakespearean presentations. There was no doubt about it, he was a talented orator and a well-respected actor. Apart from his constant bouts of ill health, due again to his breathing problems, he was enjoying the beginnings of what would surely be a successful and rewarding career.

Speechless

As his popularity began to grow and he was called upon more and more to give his one-man show, he began to suffer from a complaint that seemed utterly disastrous for an actor – he lost his voice.

The first few times it happened he was able to rest for a day or two and, when he had recovered his voice, he could continue with his shows. But the problem not only persisted – it actually began to get worse. He tried all the usual remedies of doctor's prescriptions and throat medicine but nothing seemed to work. The more shows he did, the worse his voice got. He went to various voice teachers and doctors and the only cure was complete rest.

He gave up speaking completely, on one doctor's advice, for two weeks. At the end of the fortnight his voice was back to normal and he gave a show that evening. Half-way through the show his voice went completely and he was forced to abandon the performance. The same doctor recommended that this time he give up speaking for a month. Alexander was not impressed. 'Surely,' he asked, 'if my voice was all right at the beginning of the show but let me down half-way through then it must have been something I was doing that caused it to go?' The doctor thought he might well be right but was unable to offer any further help.

The manner of doing

Alexander took to watching himself in a mirror as he rehearsed to see if there was anything he was doing that was causing the voice loss. He knew his ordinary speaking voice was not affected – it was only when he was reciting that the voice loss was triggered. He watched himself in the mirror as he spoke normally and again as he recited. He noticed that while he spoke normally nothing much happened, but that just before he began to recite he did three things: he tensed his neck causing his head to go back, he tightened his throat muscles, and he took a short deep breath. As he recited he noticed that he did these three things constantly, even exaggerating them quite wildly at times as the passion of his acting overtook him. But this was how he had been trained to project his voice as a professional actor. He found that even when he spoke normally he was still doing these three things but on a much smaller scale, he just hadn't been able to see it before (see Figure 1.1)

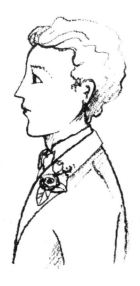

Alexander relaxing before
the show

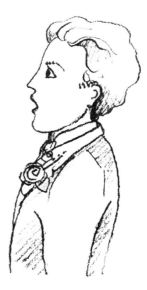

Alexander about
to begin reciting

Figure 1.1   F M Alexander noticing his problem

These observations, of what he called his *manner of doing*, became quite detailed. He used several mirrors to surround himself so he could see exactly what it was that he was doing from every angle.

Once he had seen his manner of doing he thought, quite rightly, that if he was able to stop doing the three things then his voice must improve. And he thought it would be easy to stop doing them. But he was wrong. He managed to stop tensing his neck but when he tried to control the tightening of his throat muscles or the sharp intake of breath just before he began to recite, he was unable to break the habit.

Not doing

Unable to correct his habits he was unable to rectify the problem. He decided that he would take it one step at a time, beginning with the neck tensing because he found he could control this – and this is where he made the discovery that was to lead to the Alexander Technique. He found that if he didn't tense his neck and stopped trying to correct the other two faults they disappeared on their own. By *not doing* he managed to do. He realised that by not doing he was making a conscious choice to do. This is the basic fundamental principle behind all of his subsequent teaching. This choice, he reasoned, was responsible for the quality of his performance. He called this capability of choice, *use*.

As he practised *not doing*, his voice improved and he was able to work normally. He wanted to take this discovery further and practised putting his head forwards, as he had observed that by tensing his neck it was pulled backwards. He thought that if he put his head forwards he might improve his voice even more. Whilst doing this he noticed, in his mirrors, that as soon as he put his head forwards he again tightened his throat muscles causing his larynx to constrict, and he also lifted his chest, narrowing his back which made him physically shorter. By merely putting his head forwards he changed his entire body shape and tension.

Primary control

He realised that this tension throughout his body influenced everything about him. His voice was not the problem, how he stood was not the cause, and trying to correct it all was not the cure. What he had to learn to do was *not* to do. He knew that if he put his head up and forwards he could maintain his acting voice indefinitely. All he had to do was not tense anything. Again he used mirrors to make sure he was doing exactly what he wanted to and this was when he made his second most important discovery. By observing himself he realised that when he *thought* he was putting his head up and forwards he was actually not doing that. He was still pulling it back.

He knew he had to do two things: *prevent* the movement backwards and *do* the movement forwards. But the more he tried, the harder it seemed to become. It was easy in theory but impossible in practice. The more he tried to do, the worse it became. He realised that the head position dominated the entire body attitude – but he couldn't seem to be able to move his head as he wanted to. He also saw that his head was invariably not where he thought it was. He realised that the relationship between head, neck and body influences the entire body posture and position. He called this relationship *primary control*.

Trusting his feelings

He was fascinated by these discoveries and began to apply them to all aspects of his life. He watched himself walking, standing, talking, gesturing and so on. All movements he noticed were influenced by his head position – when it was unbalanced or wrong then his entire body was tensed badly. However, he couldn't tell when it was right just by feeling or thought. He could see it physically in the mirrors but what he saw as wrong often, if not always, *felt* right. And when it felt wrong to him it looked right in the mirror.

He realised that he had developed certain habits of holding his head in a particular way for so long that it had become an unconscious trait. And this trait or habit felt right *because* he had been doing it for so long. The correct head placement felt wrong because it was new and unaccustomed. It dawned on him that he couldn't trust his feelings about where and how he was holding his body. This quite shocked him and seems, even now, to unsettle some of the basic assumptions we make about our lives. If we can't trust our perceptions of where we are and what we are doing, then what can we trust? Alexander decided that it must be possible to restore the trust. If *doing* was wrong then he would have to look more closely at *not doing*.

Inhibition

As he watched and tried to change he made another important discovery: the habit was always stronger than the desire to change. It seemed as though he only had to think about doing something before all the old habits kicked in automatically and he would tense something somewhere that he didn't want to tense.

Again he made a discovery that was to influence his future teachings. He realised that if, just as he was about to do something, he let go of the thought of doing it, then nothing tensed. He called this letting go of the thought of doing something, *inhibition*. Basically it is inhibiting the habit caused by the thought.

——— Putting it all together ———

Alexander began to put all the discoveries together. He practised at first just reciting one sentence and, as he did so, bringing into play the things he had learnt from observation:

1 Inhibiting the immediate response to speak and thus stopping the habits at source;
2 Consciously projecting the primary control directions for the improved 'use of self' which were: letting the neck be free, letting the head go forwards and up, and allowing the back to lengthen and widen;
3 To continue these directions even while speaking;
4 Just at the moment of speaking stopping again to reconsider the decision, allowing the freedom *not to speak* or to do something else.

Putting it all together certainly seemed to work. His recitals became better than ever. He found he was more relaxed, his temper corrected and his overall health was greatly improved.

───── Psychophysical integrity ─────

As he put what he had learnt into practice throughout his entire daily life he couldn't help but feel fantastic. He had found a way of managing his body to such an extent that he was in good health, relaxed, and moving with a new grace and lightness that he would never have thought possible before. He realised he had beaten his unconscious habits and learnt a new method of being which he called *psychophysical integrity*.

His performances went from being good to verging on the brilliant. His voice had improved to such an extent that he quickly gained a reputation as one of the foremost Shakespearean actors of his time.

Within a short time he was anxious to pass on his experiences. As people couldn't help but notice the dramatic improvements that he had undergone they were as anxious to learn this new discovery as he was to teach it. He soon found he had a new, additional career as a voice teacher.

───────── The work ─────────

As well as continuing his acting career and teaching voice lessons, Alexander pursued his investigations into the way humans move and operate. He called this *the work* and it was to become his passion and direction for over fifty years.

His observations led him on the next step which was to realise that the:

> so-called 'mental' and 'physical' are not separate entities and that for this reason human ills and shortcomings cannot be classified as 'mental' or 'physical' and dealt with specifically as such, but that all training, whether it be educative or otherwise, i.e. whether its object be the prevention or elimination of defect, error or disease, must be based upon the indivisible unity of the human organism.

He quickly developed a considerable following, not only amongst actors and would-be actors who wanted to develop their talent, but also from people sent to him by doctors. The medical profession may have been sceptical at first but Alexander could produce results. Principally he dealt with speech problems but, gradually, he began to see, and treat, a whole range of physical defects.

Slowly he was developing the work into the Alexander Technique. He deliberately chose not to use words and terms that might confuse his clients if they had a preconceived idea of what those terms might mean. He settled for 'the self' and 'in use' rather than 'subconscious' and 'body mechanics'.

The hands-on approach

Whilst all this might seem to have developed quickly, Alexander had actually spent nearly ten years on his work. He started to teach in earnest and found quite often that people didn't understand what he was trying to demonstrate when he merely talked to them about his work. It became a natural next step to show his audience his theories by using his hands to gently move their bodies into the right positions. This use of the hands became, and still is today, a fundamental principle of the Alexander Technique but – and this is important – it is not essential. Alexander himself learnt his work through trial and error with nobody using their hands on him. This book will teach you the Technique without you having to spend the same length of time that Alexander did in front of a mirror.

By the turn of the century he was practising in Sydney and had met, and won over, the famous surgeon, Steward McKay. McKay suggested that Alexander really should go to London if he wanted his work to gain the recognition it deserved. Alexander put on a last farewell tour of *Hamlet* and *The Merchant of Venice*, employing cured patients rather than actors, and then set sail for London in 1904.

Man's Supreme Inheritance

Once settled in London Alexander returned to acting at the same time as setting up a practice to teach his work. Within a few years he was known as 'the protector of the London theatre' and could count most of the famous actors of the day amongst his clients, including Sir Henry Irving, and he subsequently instructed the then current

Archbishop of Canterbury, as well as Aldous Huxley, Lewis Mumford, George Bernard Shaw, Henry James and many other eminent people. Nineteen doctors signed a letter to *The Lancet* urging that his Technique become recognised and evaluated by their profession because of its remarkable effectiveness in treating many of their patients.

By 1910 there was sufficient interest for unscrupulous people to set up rival practices claiming to teach the Alexander Technique. Alexander wrote and had published his first book on the subject, *Man's Supreme Inheritance*, in an attempt to set the record straight. This book was to remain in print for the rest of his life.

Off to America

With the outbreak of war in 1914 Alexander took himself off to America where he founded a new practice and for the next decade he spent half the year in America and half in London. His technique was well received and within a short time he had developed a considerably thriving business. Alexander himself was never reluctant to promote his work – his early theatrical training meant that he was still the showman. He was even accused of 'cultism' while in America – an unfounded accusation but understandable because he was the one and only teacher. However, that was to be rectified within a few years.

The first school

The first school was not for people wanting to learn how to teach the Alexander Technique but for small children. In 1924 Alexander set up an infants' school in his studio in London for children from three to eight, with the intention of teaching them proper *use of self* from an early age. This school ran until it had to be transferred to America in 1940 where it continued to thrive.

The first teacher

The first school for teachers was set up by Alexander in London in 1930, offering a three-year training course. He was absolutely resolute that anyone wanting to teach his work first had to demonstrate that they had learnt, and could exercise, proper use of themselves. Alexander's brother, Albert Alexander, was probably his first trainee teacher. Albert had broken his back in a riding accident and had been told he would never walk again. Alexander taught him about *inhibition*, *primary control* and *conscious direction*. Albert practised in his hospital bed until he was up and moving about. Less than two years after his paralysing accident he was fully recovered and a walking example of the effectiveness of the Technique. He was to remain a lifelong teacher, follower, and exponent.

Libel

Alexander's first infant school teacher was Irene Tasker who ran the school for ten years, until she emigrated to South Africa in 1934 where she set up the first independent practice. She had qualified as an Alexander Teacher and, with Alexander's approval, was determined to spread the work as wide and as far as possible. This included trying to get it placed on the curriculum of physical education throughout South African schools. The director of the South African Physical Education Committee, Dr Ernst Jokl, was not a devotee, however, and he launched a particularly offensive attack on Alexander who was left with no choice except to sue for libel.

The case dragged on for many years until, in 1948, Alexander won. The strain of the trial, which he had been unable to attend in person, left him exhausted – he was now nearly eighty – and he suffered a stroke. This was to prove an even greater test than curing his loss of voice. He naturally used his own Technique on himself and within a few weeks was back teaching and working. He lived for another seven years and died in 1955, aged 86. Not a bad length of life for someone written off as weak and sickly as a child and unable even to attend school.

Spreading the word

During Alexander's lifetime the success of the Alexander Technique was clearly demonstrated. Many eminent doctors and scientists came forward to attest to its remarkable successes. Famous people took lessons and reported widely how effective and reliable it was. On the surface it was a truly extraordinary new development in body awareness and should have attracted a wider following than it did. Part of the reason it didn't was Alexander's own personality. He was not a therapist as we would understand it today – he didn't suffer fools gladly and was quite a tyrant when it came to following the standards he set.

He was also not a conformist and cared little for society. He even moved his mistress into his home with his wife and cared nothing for the scandal it created. He was an inveterate gambler and his love of horseracing sometimes threatened to overshadow his work. He was even declared bankrupt over a debt. He was a forceful person who liked the best that money could buy – good food and fine wines. There was even something of the dandy about him. At times he was dismissed as brash and loud, but he didn't ever attempt to modify or tone down his behaviour. He was a strong individualist and there's no doubt he upset a lot of people. However, viewed with hindsight, he would have fared better in today's climate of media attention and his Technique would have made it on to many a good chat show.

—— The Alexander Technique today ——

Since Alexander's death his Technique has gone on quietly growing in strength. Many famous people still attest to its quality, and it is taught in schools and colleges. There are many qualified Alexander Technique teachers, a governing body and a wide following throughout the world. Today you can go to a teacher and have personal lessons, learn about it in books like this one, attend group introductory seminars and listen to Alexander cassettes. The Technique's applications are many and varied. It used to be seen as something actors or musicians did to relieve stress and tensions but slowly it has spread as a personal body awareness which teaches you how to manage and use your body well. It is also used as a preventive for many body defects such as backache and Repetitive Strain Injury.

Because the Technique is such a personal thing with sometimes small demonstrable effects it can become overshadowed by more dramatic therapies and it is probably the most misunderstood of the therapies available – even Alexander himself was hard pushed to come up with a suitable definition, or perhaps he chose not to.

With or without a physical defect to correct, you can learn and benefit from the Alexander Technique purely because it's a method of coping with the unnatural stresses we put upon the human frame by the demands of civilised living. This was something Alexander himself was very aware of. Once, when explaining his work to his father, his father asked why we should need to learn anything like it when animals managed to perform their physical activities perfectly naturally. Alexander explained that if animals were expected to do half the things we were in a civilised society then they too would need attention. We place unbearable burdens on our bodies by the way we live and, because we grow up with the habit of burden, we don't even realise it – it has come to feel right. We sit in chairs, drive cars, watch TV, use stairs, indulge in 'sports', and carry out a million and one unnatural acts that animals don't.

Summary

Alexander developed his Technique as a result of his own problems of voice loss. He saw the cause as threefold:

- he tensed his neck causing his head to go back
- he tightened his throat muscles
- he took a short deep breath.

He also developed some fundamental principles that can be summed up as:

- *the manner of doing* – how we develop the habits that precede movements;
- *not doing* – the more we try to correct the faults, the worse we can make it; by not doing we can learn more;
- *primary control* – the relationship between head, neck and torso influences the entire body;
- *inhibiting* – old habits are stronger than the desire to change; before movement we have a choice whether we begin the movement or not.

I expect you'll be anxious to get on and see how all this can affect you. Before you rush ahead – what Alexander called *end gaining* (we'll learn more about that shortly) – try the following exercises and see if any of the things Alexander discovered apply to you.

EXERCISES

These exercises are not tests. There is no right or wrong. They are merely designed to get you thinking about how you hold your body. Don't worry if it all feels uncomfortable and new – we'll sort it all out in the next few chapters.

1 While you are sitting reading this try folding your arms as you would do normally. How does it feel? Comfortable and relaxed? Now try folding your arms the opposite way – if you normally fold left over right try right over left. Now how does it feel? Even if you managed to do it quite easily – and I doubt that since most people find it quite difficult to swop arms – how does it feel now? Awkward and uncomfortable? Does one shoulder feel higher than the other? When you fold your arms normally one shoulder has to be higher and comfortable. Doing it the other way round is neither better nor worse, right or wrong, it's just different. But because it is not a habit it feels awkward.

2 Now try standing up. Without looking stand with your feet parallel and about 30 cm (12 inches) apart. Now look down and see how accurate you were. Try doing it when you haven't had time to think about it – it's quite common to be either not parallel, or further apart or closer together than you think.

3 Try standing next to a full length mirror. Without looking in it (keep your eyes closed) adopt a position that feels comfortable. You don't have to stand up straight or anything like that – the Alexander Technique is not about that – just relax and stand comfortably. You don't have to be facing the mirror. Now open your eyes and look carefully at yourself. Are you looking as comfortable as you feel? Does your posture appear as relaxed and easy as you thought it was with your eyes closed?

4 Just before you begin to do something – and it could be anything like filling the kettle, getting out of bed, being about to eat something, cleaning your teeth, waving to a friend across the street – stop before you do it and freeze. Now mentally check your body posture, especially your head and neck. Are you already craning forwards to begin the task? Have you tensed muscles you won't need? Does the position you've frozen in feel comfortable? Could you now decide not to do what you were going to? Could you now do something else? Could you hold the position you're now in for a while or would it quickly become uncomfortable?

2

WHAT IS THE THE ALEXANDER TECHNIQUE?

You translate everything, whether physical, mental or spiritual, into muscular tension.

F M Alexander

The Society of Teachers of the Alexander Technique (STAT) has this to say about the Alexander Technique:

> when the natural subconscious mechanisms for balance and posture are disturbed by habitual misuse or injury the standard of our physical and mental functioning can be adversely affected. However, the appropriate muscular activity for posture is not something we can regain by simply trying harder. It involves 'automatic' reflex responses that, when working well, appear to support the body almost effortlessly.

Basically, we have not learnt how to adapt our bodies to modern living – it took a million years for us to adapt to living as humans and we've had only the last 100 000 years to get used to being civilised. It's not long enough. Added to this is the way we are brought up. How many times have you heard 'stand up straight', 'sit up straight', 'sit still, don't fidget!' So, when you were a small child, how did you stand up straight? Usually you threw your shoulders back, stuck out your chest as far as possible and curved your spine. Didn't you? (Figure 2.1)

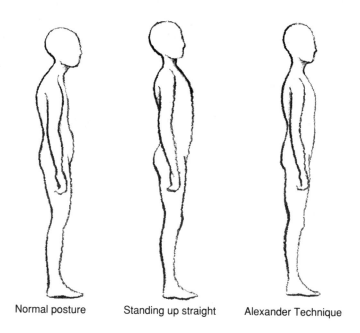

Normal posture   Standing up straight   Alexander Technique

Figure 2.1   Standing up straight

And how do you sit up straight? Again by adopting a tensed position that you think is straight but when viewed from the side is very peculiar (see Figure 2.2)

And as for sitting still – well, you could if the chairs were designed for human beings. Unfortunately they're not – or rather human beings are not designed for chairs. Chairs haven't been around long enough for us to evolve into them. If you watch any of the native people of Australia or South America you will observe a natural grace and ease of movement – but you won't see any chairs, or a whole range of modern equipment that is supposed to make our lives easier. And no, don't go throwing away all your furniture before you've finished reading this book. At the end of it you can choose to do so if you wish. The Alexander Technique is about choices. We sit in chairs because we believe we have no choice, that's all there is to it. And that's partly right. We also sit down and stand up in a certain way because that's the way we do it – we believe we have no choice.

The Alexander Technique will give you an alternative. Once learnt you will have choice – conscious choice – in everything you do for the rest of your life. You may still choose to throw your furniture away if you want. You may also claim you can't remember all that you've learnt about the Alexander Technique – and *that's* your choice.

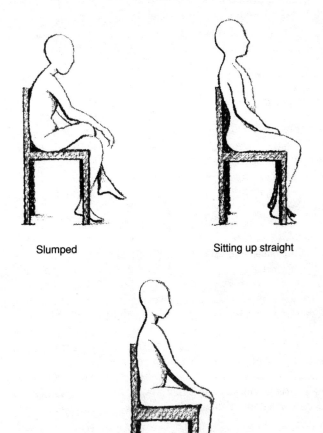

Slumped   Sitting up straight

Alexander Technique

Figure 2.2   Sitting up straight

——— The fundamental things ———

What I would like to do now is go through with you some of the technical terms and how they apply. This isn't complicated or difficult – it's just that Alexander liked to use new terminology for some of his principles so that there would be no confusion. Some of these terms are, by their very nature, unfamiliar but they are quite easy to understand – we have already met some of them for the first time in the previous chapter.

Primary control

Alexander rightly observed that the relationship between the head, neck and torso affects the whole body. If the head and neck are properly aligned with the back, then the whole body naturally follows into a relaxed, natural posture. The problem is that we don't know what properly aligned is – we have never learnt it – and this is probably the vital learning aspect of the Alexander Technique. This problem seems to affect only humans. Are we a design fault? Have we evolved badly? Look at any of the other mammals: cats flow smoothly as they walk; monkeys swing gracefully through the trees; dolphins swim in a perfect streamlined way; leopards run effortlessly. Look at humans and we seem a misconstructed bunch. We sag and walk badly, ache and become unfit. Are we designed to walk on all fours? Or upright on two legs? Left to our own devices we might well spend a lot of the time closer to the ground. We would squat rather than sit in chairs, lounge around on the floor rather than slump on sofas. If you watch children they tend to gravitate towards the floor on most occasions. Parents are forever telling them to 'get up off the floor' as if they're likely to catch some dreadful disease if they lie on the carpet – and yet all they are doing is being, quite naturally, natural.

If you watch soldiers on parade they stand up straight. They are our finest fighting people and should be at their peak of physical fitness. Yet if you watch them they appear stiff and ill-at-ease.

Alexander said that the head should be directed up and forwards. This direction is not done by deliberately pushing the head into that position but by *consciously projecting*. Once the head is properly aligned the rest of the body follows (see Figure 2.3).

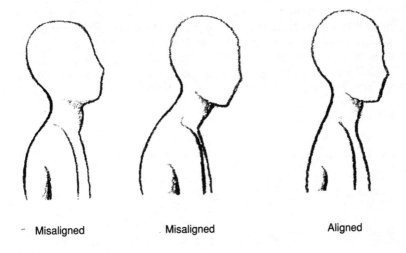

| Misaligned | Misaligned | Aligned |

Figure 2.3 The alignment of the head

You can see from Figure 2.1 that there are different ways of standing. When we try to stand up straight, or properly, or according to our ideas of 'right', we invariably alter the position of our back, chest or upper torso in some way. Alexander realised that the head leads the entire body posture. Get the head right and the rest will follow suit. Get the head wrong and you'll never be able to do much with the rest of it. However, getting the head right is the most difficult thing to achieve. The reason why most Alexander teachers suggest, quite importantly, that you need lessons on a one-to-one basis is for just that reason – to get the head right.

What's right and what's wrong?

I talk about 'right' and 'wrong' as if there is some overall correct head position. There isn't. There is a right position for you and you alone. We all have different bodies, different heads and different ways of standing, walking, sitting and lying down. To get the head right for all of us using only one position is impossible. All we can attempt to do is get it right for ourselves.

The word *right* is not right. When we talk about right we usually mean good or correct. With the Alexander Technique there is no such thing as 'right' or 'wrong'. There is a *better* position for the head to be in which will allow the rest of the body to become free – but there is no right or wrong. You may well know which position is better for you, you may know full well how to achieve it, and yet you can still choose to stand in a 'wrong' way. Again the whole basis is choice. Something can be wrong only if we do it because we have no choice. Once we have choice we can stand however we like.

How to achieve primary control

EXERCISE

Close your eyes and imagine that there is a string attached to the top of your head and it is pulling you gently upright. Just sit for a moment imagining this. As you do so I want you to feel exactly what is happening to your body. I expect you will have imperceptibly moved your head upwards. Your back may have straightened and you will have pulled yourself upright.

However, the instruction was to *imagine* what the string was doing.

Now try again knowing, this time, that no body movement is necessary. Just imagine what is happening without moving. Alexander was well aware of the extremely powerful links there are between mind and body. Primary control starts in the mind. If you give your mind an instruction it will subtly control your body.

During the next few days constantly, in different situations, imagine the string pulling you gently upwards. You don't have to do anything. Allow your mind to work on the body at a very subconscious level.

Conscious projection

Alexander, being aware of the close relationship between mind and body, reasoned that if you reprogramed the mind, the body would automatically follow. However, the reprograming is the hardest part. Alexander suggested that the way to do it was to repeat constantly specific instructions so that we can hear them as we were moving. The problem with this is that you soon quickly learn to stop listening – you start to treat the mental directions like a kind of mantra, then you start to feel it is of no value and stop doing it. However, as anyone who has ever used a mantra to meditate will know, the mind operates on a very subtle level. Things are happening when we don't even notice.

Alexander's conscious projections were:

● let the neck be free
● let the head go forwards and up
● allow the back to lengthen and widen.

Again these are not things for you to *do* – they are thoughts for you to think. They are *conscious projections*. You *can* use them like a mantra: repeat them whenever you have a moment to spare; repeat them whenever you sit down, stand up, walk, move, gesture. And every time you find that you are moving as you mentally recite the conscious projection then you should stop and remember that they are only thoughts not actions. We have the thoughts first and the actions follow automatically. There is no need for us to *do* anything. In fact, as Alexander found out – and it took him about ten years – the more we try to do the worse we will make things.

End gaining

How can trying to do something make it worse? Well, you're being given permission to do nothing. The reason that we let our bodies get into the state that they are in is because we are all doers. Doing causes the problems. When we let go and stop doing we benefit. Not doing is probably the most difficult thing we can do. Humans are great at doing. We build cities, travel to the stars, explore remote continents, climb mountains and drive cars. You name it, we do it. In fact the Hopi Indians of America call Westerners the 'termite people'. We do so much. Here's a conversation from your childhood:

PARENT: [*to child in another room*] What are you doing?
CHILD: Nothing.
PARENT: Well come here and I'll find you something to do.
CHILD: But I'm happy doing nothing at the moment.
PARENT: That's no way to spend your time. You ought to be doing something!

Maybe it's not exactly how you heard it, but it'll be similar. And when we become parents ourselves we forget those childhood delights of doing absolutely nothing. We too tell our children to do something.

This constant doing has created many habits in us. Whenever we have to do something we concentrate on *what* we have to do and not on the *way* in which we do it. End gaining is probably best observed

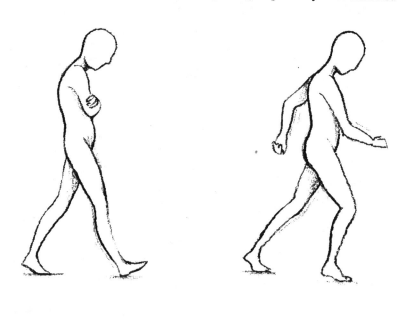

Figure 2.4   Examples of end gaining in action

in people in a hurry – maybe they are rushing to catch a train. Their heads will be down and forwards with the rest of the body following on behind at a considerable angle (see Figure 2.4).

Figure 2.4 is an extreme example, but we end gain in every aspect of our lives, some worse than others. I have to admit to a particular over-indulgence myself. Once, when I was at college, I took a break for coffee. The coffee shop was just across the road. Just outside the coffee shop was a lamp post. I had passed it every day for three years. I had walked round it, seen it, noticed it – I knew it was there. But I wanted coffee. I end gained my way to the coffee shop at such a pace that I ran straight into the lamp post and knocked myself out. End gaining can be painful. I knew that the lamp post was there but I just didn't see it. I was concentrating so hard on my objective that I missed the journey entirely. How many other journeys have I missed?

EXERCISE

I expect you've seen the street or road where you live many times. You've seen your front door many times. But I bet you've always seen it while you've been end gaining. Next time you come home from work I want you to try and notice something about your front entrance that you've never seen before. Try this exercise over several days. You probably won't run out of things to notice – they're there, just like the lamp post, but we've been too busy getting our keys out to open the door, thinking about what we're going to have for supper, worrying about whether we've missed the news or not, planning tomorrow, planning our evening, planning the rest of our lives. You name it and we're doing it. All I want you to do is take a little time to look around for once – you can do all the other stuff later.

After you've done this for a few days I want you to go back to end gaining – it's a conscious choice so it's not wrong. Now compare how you felt physically while you were end gaining and not end gaining.

Looking around to notice new things makes us more relaxed. We walk with more grace because we're not being head-led. We're not rushing forwards. And yet we'll still move at the same speed. We lose nothing. By not end gaining, we gain.

Try not end gaining in your living room, or garden. Stroll around noticing things you may never have seen before. Walk to the shops and instead of thinking about what you're going to buy, try to look around and enjoy the journey.

End gaining in action

End gaining can be seen in every aspect of our society. The end result is always the most important. We have to get results, and it doesn't matter what we do to ourselves to get those results. It starts as soon as we go to school. Getting exam results is important. We have to look to the future. But I wonder if the quality of our children's education suffers because of end gaining. We rarely seem to think of how we learn – it's always learning to achieve a result. The scenario seems to be to pass exams so we can go on to higher education to gain a qualification that will enable us to hold down a good job that will see us being promoted higher and higher, because as we rise higher we earn more money and earning more money produces results because we will be happier. Unfortunately for many people, this scenario simply doesn't work. They may end up with the exam, the job, the promotion and even the money – but often it's the happiness they have somehow missed out on. End gaining is something we all do. Learning how to stop is the key. And we learn by unlearning.

End gaining in our lives

You may like to spend some time working out your own examples of end gaining. How do you rush ahead? We all think to next year's holiday and then when we're on holiday, we think ahead to going back to work.

End gaining is a mental attitude – rushing ahead without enjoying the journey. But, as Alexander knew, the mental affects the physical. When we *unlearn* end gaining we can be more relaxed. We'll still arrive, it'll still take the same time to arrive, but maybe we won't be quite so frazzled when we do get there. And this applies to every aspect of our lives from the smallest task or journey to the really big things in life, like life and death itself.

The 'means whereby'

End gaining is a habit. Maybe it was once a necessary habit to allow us to survive in caves or when hunting. This habit can be unlearnt, but we need to take apart every movement we make and see why we move like it. Alexander called this analysis the *means whereby*. How do we *do*? We do by the 'means whereby'. Each action has a means whereby. As we sit, or stand up again, we have a means whereby. Once we start to look at each action needed to complete a task we can begin to question various factors:

- **How am I doing this task** – What muscles am I using? How is my body placed? How does it feel? How do the different parts of my body feel in relation to all the other parts?
- **Why am I doing this task** – What is the end gain? What will be the result after I have done this task? Why should I continue to do this task? What motivates me to do this task? Is this task suitable for me to do?

EXERCISE

While you're reading this, you might as well make good use of your time. Without moving a single part of you, I want you to mentally do a stock take of your body. Start with your feet and work your way up. I want you to monitor each part of your anatomy. Where is it? What's it doing? How's it feel? What's it touching? Is it tense or relaxed? What does it look like in your mind's eye? What does your whole body look like? What does it feel like?

You got yourself into this position, now I want to know how you got there and why? Why are your fingers placed just so? Why are your feet where they are? Where is your head and why? Monitor every-thing – but move nothing at this stage.

By now you'll probably be acutely aware that certain parts are in strange positions. You're gradually waking up to the fact that your body seems to have arrived somewhere without you having had anything to do with it. Don't worry, this is a normal part of the Alexander Technique. It's as if we suddenly find ourselves inhabit-ing a strange container that has a will of its own.

Now you know where all the parts are – and you haven't moved any of them – I want you to complete part two of this exercise. Start to plan where you would put all the parts – again without moving – if you'd consciously been aiming to sit more comfortably, or more relaxed, or better. Again don't move, but prepare yourself mentally first.

Part three is for you to stand up now and give yourself time to get ready to sit down again and continue reading. Practise the con-scious projection as you prepare yourself. Just before you sit again try to remember where all the parts were and which ones you had decided to change. It may be a bit like being in bed just before you fall asleep; you've found a really comfortable position but then you suddenly have to go to the bathroom. When you return you can't quite remember how it was that you felt so comfortable, and it feels uncomfortable until you settle again. The newness of a posi-tion can sometimes feel awkward because it's not habit.

This exercise can be done at any time, in any place. Whatever you find yourself doing, just stop and monitor all the parts and repeat the exercise.

Alexander urged his pupils to concentrate on the 'means of the doing', not on the end gain, and by so doing they would naturally relax and move better. When we fail to question the means whereby we are acting like automatons. When we analyse the means whereby we start to move like human beings: we are in control and taking responsibility, we are making conscious choices.

Inhibitions

This is Alexander's word for learning to stop just before beginning to do or move. It has come to mean other things since his time, but we will use the word as he meant it – learning to stop.

It's not just about learning to stop, it's about learning to stop to question what we are doing and the means whereby we are going to do it. Inhibition is also an excellent way to avoid end gaining. If every time you are about to rush at something you inhibit first, it gives you a chance to pause to draw breath – to take a little time to become conscious of what you are doing. You can then check the motivation for the task, how it's to be done, what will happen if it's done and how you feel about doing it. These things take only a fraction of a second to do – it's not as if you need to sit down and ponder laboriously for hours, it's just that tiny pause before action while you check that you still want to go ahead.

EXERCISE

You will need a pen and paper for this. I want you to write down exactly how you do three everyday things:

1 How do you get dressed in the mornings? In what order do you put on your clothes? How do you stand or sit while you're doing it? Now I want you to explain, in writing, why you do it like this. You're not allowed to rehearse first – do this from memory;
2 How do you go to sleep at night? How do you get into bed? In what position do you lie? Where exactly is every part of your body? And again, why do you do it like this?
3 How do you make tea/coffee? What do you do while the kettle is boiling? How do you stand? Where is everything positioned? Why?

That's all quite easy, isn't it? Or did you find it hard to remember exactly what you do? It doesn't matter because later on you're going to do part two of this exercise. Put the paper with your details to one side and, when the time comes to do these activities, you can check against your details to see how accurate you have been.

After that you can do part three of the exercise which is to repeat the activities, when they occur naturally, and this time inhibit before each and every action. This will give you a pause to check each action to make sure it's what you really want to do. Don't worry at this stage about whether you're doing it right or wrong – just be open to waking up to the fact that you may have been operating unconsciously all your life. The Alexander Technique is about waking up, questioning what we do, and then finding a better, more efficient, conscious method of doing.

Anti-gravity

The effects of gravity are well known by everyone. What may need to be emphasised is how permanent gravity is. It doesn't stop just because we cease to think about it. It's working twenty-four hours a day, pulling everything towards the centre of the Earth – and that includes us. Every muscle, every tendon, every fibre of our being is fighting gravity all the time. If we didn't we would be little floppy heaps on the floor. The human body is an anti-gravity entity. It is able to withstand the attacks gravity makes on it for the whole of its life. However, the price that we have to pay is pretty high. Over the years the battle leaves us saggy and stooped. We get beaten down – never defeated – but we can look and feel war-worn and scarred.

Alexander suggests that we could help ourselves become more efficient anti-gravity devices if we were aware of what was going on and had a little help. He knew the mind is pretty powerful so suggested that we could imagine the string attached to our heads pulling us upright. That string is free from gravity (because it's imaginary) and thus could keep us more upright without losing it's efficiency. If you want to be convinced about the power of the mind just think about your name – it is you, it has a shape and an identity, you write it, people know you by it, you have had it all your life, it is an undeniable part of you and all you represent. Correct? Yes. But it has no reality – it doesn't actually exist. If something that doesn't exist has that much power, what can you do if you start to use that power consciously and constructively?

Function

Each part of our body has function. This function is part of its inherent design. The function and its related design are specifically geared to complete certain tasks. Some body parts have function that is obvious and cannot easily be misused – take your ears for instance. They are ears, they do hearing things and rarely can we use them for anything else. Now take your back. What's its function? What is it actually for? To support the upper part of your body? To lift heavy things? Something clever God thought of to hang the arms on?

In Chapter 8 we will look more closely at the human body, its components and their function. At the moment it's enough to know that every part has function – and every part has potential function misuse. If we don't know what the correct function is, we cannot correct any misuse.

Stimuli

Suppose someone, a close friend, whom you know really well and respect, comes into the room. They look at you and tell you that they find you stupid, unattractive and rather a waste of space. Imagine how you would react. They've given you the stimulus, now you can have the reaction. You'd probably burst into tears or run away or shout at them – all of these actions are physical manifestations of stimuli. But remember inhibition. You could take time out to inhibit before you react – and then choose how you will react. You may, having thought about it, choose to not react at all. Your friend smiles broadly and explains it was a joke, a test, they were drunk, whatever.

Suppose every time the 'phone rings you jump up to answer it. Suppose you're in the middle of something really important – a good argument or making love or having supper – and the 'phone rings. The stimulus is the ringing sound; what's your response? Most people, not knowing about inhibiting, still jump up and answer it. Now you know about inhibiting you can take a tiny fraction of a second just to question whether what you're doing may be more important – and continue doing it. Besides which, the answering machine can always react for you, if you have one.

Stimulus is anything which spurs us into action. It could be: emotional – every time we hear a particular piece of music we feel sad; physical – the 'phone ringing makes us jump up; mental – every time I think about all the work I have to do my brain goes cloudy.

Some stimuli set off reactions that are learnt habits and are very difficult not to respond to. I bet we all look when we hear a police siren. We know it's nothing to do with us but we still react whether we want to or not. Sometimes these stimuli are very important, even life saving. In a theatre if someone shouts 'fire' then we need to react. But now we know about inhibiting we maybe don't need to panic – instead we can choose a more productive response.

Summary

In this chapter we have looked at some of the important terms associated with the Alexander Technique and what they mean:

- primary control
- conscious projection
- end gaining
- the means whereby
- inhibitions
- anti-gravity
- function
- stimuli.

If any of these still feel unfamiliar to you or you're not sure exactly what they mean, it might be worth re-reading this chapter. These terms will be used a lot in later chapters and it will help if you have become easy with them.

As there have been plenty of exercises during this chapter I guess you can be let off homework for once – but I want you ready for chapter 3 first thing in the morning!

3
WHAT'S IT FOR?

You get what you 'feel' is the right position, but that only means that you're getting the position which fits in with your defective co-ordination.

F M Alexander

As humans evolved it was a necessary part of the process to evolve certain defence mechanisms at the same time. The human body, especially the head with its valuable contents, is a very delicate and sensitive piece of equipment that must be protected at all costs. When we lived in caves we had certain responses to danger – responses we still have to this day. These responses are triggered by external stimuli, such as a wild animal approaching, or internal stimuli – body sensors such as the pain response that tell us if we are falling over or need protecting in some other way.

Flight or fight?

When these responses are triggered unnecessarily we develop stress patterns that cause muscular tensions throughout the body. The old 'flight or fight' response we developed is still part of our human make up, but it is not used nearly as much as it once was. However, we still react to potential danger in the same ways we always have – it's just no longer socially acceptable to fight our enemies physically, or indeed to run away.

Falling down people

So what do we do with all the defence mechanisms the body brings into play when we think we are being threatened? Usually we store them in the form of muscular stress – tensions we learn to live with. And it's the same with the internal stimuli. If, every time our body thinks it's going to fall over, it reacts by tensing and preparing itself for injury but then doesn't fall over, it will store that tension as well. The trouble is that, because of the way we have learnt to move, our body thinks it is going to fall over constantly. This chapter is about learning to recognise and eliminate those stored responses. We can't stop the body reacting, but we can change the reaction.

— Letting go of excessive tension —

Before we can let go of any excess tension we have to understand how and why we 'tensed up' and why we continue to hold that tension afterwards. It's all to do with fear. We are frightened most, if not all, of the time. I know you'll be shaking your head at this and disagreeing, so let me explain.

Nature lets us take care of ourselves by incorporating certain reflexes into us. Those reflexes have a very short 'trigger time'. In other words they sit there activated but not actually responding all the time, permanently ready to be switched on whenever there is any hint of danger. It's as if we are living our lives constantly on edge.

In some people the trigger mechanisms are very raw and you probably know people like that: they react by suddenly jumping no matter what – a 'phone rings and they physically jump. Other people have what appears to be a much more laid back response time – they don't jump so noticeably. However, they will still react.

There are certain basic symptoms of these reactions. They are usually called the 'startle pattern' and they can be seen physically, and monitored internally (see Figure 3.1).

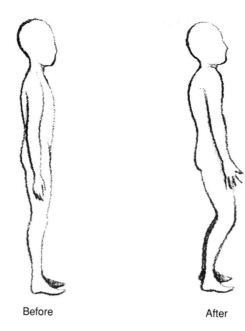

Before   After

Figure 3.1   The startle pattern

Physical changes

- head gets pulled down and back
- shoulders raise and hunch
- chest flattens
- arms straighten
- legs bend.

Physiological changes

- blood thickens
- blood pressure increases
- pulse rate increases
- heartbeat speeds up
- digestive system shuts down
- hormones such as adrenalin are released
- arteries constrict.

There are other changes as well that could be classified in either list: lungs suck in more air, skin colour changes, temperature drops, sweat glands become activated – even hair will stand on end. All in all, radical changes take place throughout the entire human system. And it happens every time we engage the startle pattern. Can you imagine what it's doing to your body when the 'phone rings? The startle pattern obviously comes into play to a greater or lesser extent depending on our basic nature, frequency and familiarity with the stimulus, and how we have learnt to cope with stress.

Coping with stress

The Alexander Technique is about learning how we respond, and how we can change some of those responses. You might not be able to control the startle pattern when you are seriously frightened, and nor should you want to. All the body changes are very necessary in order to enable us to cope when our lives are threatened. But after the threat, real or imaginary, has departed we hold on to all that tension when we can learn to let go of it. By learning inhibition we can learn how not to respond on such an instinctive level. Taking that microsecond to evaluate the situation, do we need to react to the maximum? Or could we get away with just a little reflex panic? Should our whole system be put on red alert when the 'phone rings? Or should we save that for when the wild beasts are coming?

The body needs all the changes if we are actually to fight or run away – all that extra oxygen and blood will be put to good use, and the head retracting could save you from a mortal blow. But once the danger is passed we can let go of all the tension. By monitoring our entire system we quickly learn to recognise when we have tensed up and can then deliberately let go.

Falling down again

Obviously a lot of the time the stimuli will be external – road rage, difficult people, unpleasant situations, accidents, disasters and acts of God. But what if we were startling ourselves all the time? Well, I hate to have to be the one to tell you, but we are.

When the external stimuli affect us we can usually see what is going on, but if the stimulus is internal it's a lot more difficult to detect. What if we think we're falling down and don't even know it? All the body's defence mechanisms would come into play and all we would know is that we feel stressed or tired from excess muscular tension or even irritable because we are feeling unsettled and don't know why.

I called us 'falling down people' because most of us do spend a lot of time falling down but don't realise it. One of the principal lessons in the Alexander Technique is to do with sitting down and standing up. This can perplex students who go for lessons with a teacher. Your teacher will spend a lot of time sitting you down and standing you up and you're never quite sure why. Sometimes you seem to get it 'right', but mostly you don't. The reason so much time is devoted to sitting down and standing up is that they are activities that occupy a lot of our waking time, and they are also a good way to really get to understand how and why we tense up.

Internal sensors

Internal sensors detect where and how we are, in terms of balance and space. These sensors haven't evolved at the same pace as our civilisations so they still operate in the same way that our flight or fight responses do, on a primitive level. Basically they tell our brains what we are doing and which muscles we need to be able to do it. When we are standing up we need the big muscles in our back to hold us upright. When we are lying down those big muscles can be turned off as the body knows we are going to sleep. Some of these sensors work by picking up clues from the position of our feet. If our feet are flat on the floor we are standing up and the muscles get turned on. If our feet aren't touching the floor then we must be lying down and those muscles can be turned off. It's only a two way switch – on or off – standing up or lying down. That's it and it's simple and it works. So some dumb human had to invent chairs and confuse the whole thing. Sitting is not standing and not quite lying down. As we go to sit down we temporarily lose our balance and for a fraction of a second fall backwards. Result? Yes, all the startle pattern responses come into play and we get very tense every time we sit down to relax. No wonder we're confused.

You might wonder how we used to sit. Well, we didn't. We did what all graceful and natural people do – we squatted. This kept our feet flat on the ground so that the big back muscles stayed active and supported us.

Not falling down people

So what can we do about it? We can either stop sitting in chairs and return to squatting, or we can learn to sit down without falling down – and that's easy.

EXERCISE

Try sitting down a few times. Use a hard-backed chair like a kitchen chair. Obviously you have to stand up as many times as you sit down. Each time feel what your head and neck are doing.

Now try it with your hands placed on the back of your neck. You can just lightly rest your finger tips there and see what happens now. Does your neck go back? Can you feel yourself tensing? Most people sit by lowering themselves into the chair using their hands or arms and, just as their bottom is about to reach the chair, they let go and fall the last inch or so. This causes the startle reflex and the head goes back and all the other changes we mentioned come into play. You sit and feel worse than before – and that's why.

Try sitting by lowering yourself very slowly – keep your finger tips on the back of your neck – and imagine that someone is about to pull the chair away from under you. You should be able to stop at any moment because at no point do you 'let go'. You keep your balance and don't fall. This means you don't activate the startle reflex so there's no tension and you get to feel relaxed.

It takes some practice because the only way you're going to be able to stand up again is if you let your body fall forwards slightly. Your body will not allow itself to fall and so will propel you forwards and up.

Please study Figures 3.2 and 3.3 carefully and see how you get on.

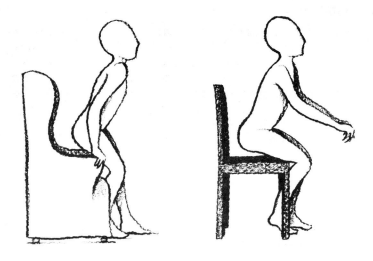

Figure 3.2　Sitting without the Alexander Technique

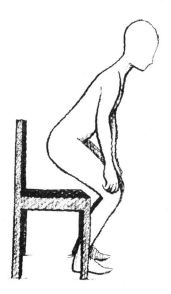

Figure 3.3　Sitting with the Alexander Technique

Couch potatoes

It's best if you do the sitting and the standing up exercise from an upright, fairly hard chair. If you try to do it from a sofa you'll have problems. If you want to extend the exercise to include sofas, you'll have to move yourself forwards, from the sitting position, to the front edge of the sofa. That way you'll be in the optimum position to 'fall' upright (see Figure 3.4).

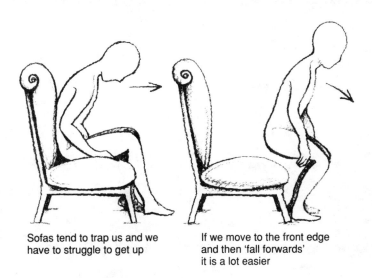

Sofas tend to trap us and we have to struggle to get up

If we move to the front edge and then 'fall forwards' it is a lot easier

Figure 3.4   Sofa sitting

Levering yourself up

This 'falling' upright can be used whenever you have to get up from a sitting position. Two activities that it's worth looking at to see how you do them are getting out of bed and getting out of a car. Again try doing them first as you would normally. Then put your finger tips at the back of your neck and try them again. The fingers on the back of the neck have two purposes: they let you feel all the tension you would normally apply as you get up; they stop you using your hands or arms to lever yourself up. Levering is what most people do when they want to get up from a sitting position.

What's standing up?

If you look at Figure 3.5 you will see that the actual percentage of the human body that needs to be altered to stand is about one third. When you're sitting down you're already two-thirds standing up. Your head, neck and torso are standing up, your lower legs are standing up, it's only your thighs that have to change position – they're the only bits sitting down. By sloping them forwards slightly you're giving them a head start and by using your head to swing yourself forwards and up you only have to pivot your thighs through about 45 degrees.

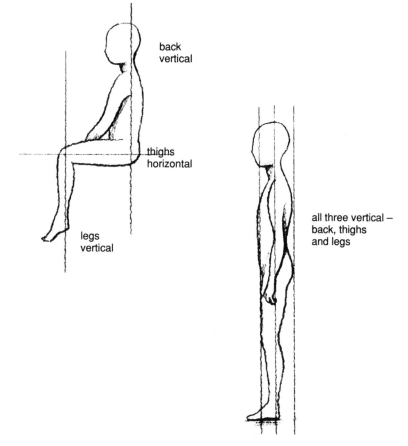

Figure 3.5   Thighs standing up ratio

Your head, neck and torso have to move forwards but not change their angle. Your feet and lower legs stay where they are. It's only your thighs that move. It's a simple operation that we all put too much effort into. We don't need to lever ourselves and we don't need to use up valuable energy using the wrong muscles to stand up or sit down.

—— The two types of muscles ——

We do in fact have the two types of muscles – voluntary (non-postural) and involuntary (postural). They have different qualities, characteristics, purposes, advantages and disadvantages.

- Voluntary muscles such as the muscles in your arms and legs are very flexible, they get exhausted quickly and they need to be directed by you. They are used for manipulation such as fetching or carrying, holding, moving and general duties. Basically they enable us to do things;
- Involuntary muscles such as the muscles you have in your back are not very flexible. They can work almost indefinitely and they are 'switched' on by the body's sensors without any input from you. They are used for maintaining the body's posture, resisting tensions and strains such as when we lift heavy objects, and changing our shape or position. Basically they hold us upright.

The two types shouldn't be confused: you use your involuntary muscles to stand up and your voluntary muscles to hold your newspaper when you want to read. You wouldn't expect the involuntary muscles in your back to do the newspaper holding for you and yet you expect the voluntary muscles in your arms to do the standing up for you.

The two systems of nerves in muscles

There are two systems of nerves in muscles. We have known about the first system for a long time; it is the system whereby the fibres in the muscles are contracted or shortened. When the nerves stop 'firing' the fibres are relaxed and the muscles lengthen again. The second system has been discovered only recently and it consists of collections of nerves that don't actually go to the muscles themselves but to lots of microscopic bundles buried deep inside the muscles called 'muscle spindles'. They lie alongside the muscle fibres and are responsible for lengthening the muscles. Previously we thought the muscles just relaxed when the first system of nerves stopped firing. Now we know that there is a second process going on as well. The second system could be likened to a fine tuning of the muscles and the spindles have little muscles of their own. They work to prevent the muscles over-contracting when we are using them – a sort of shock absorber.

Dead spindles

When we shorten our muscles continually without relaxing properly, the second system can become inactive and the spindles 'go dead'. This leads to a further shortening of the muscles and the result is poor posture and sagging body form.

The Alexander Technique is about lengthening those muscles again which in turn reactivates the muscle spindles and allows us to restore full muscle use and activity. People have often said that using the Alexander Technique leads to them feeling fitter and healthier over-all, and 'more alive'. It's often the case that because the second system of muscle nerves has been restored to life and is working again that they feel generally better.

Growing taller

Research by Dr W Barlow with fifty students at the Royal College of Music in London showed dramatic improvements when they were taught the Alexander Technique. After only 6 months 49 of them had increased their height by up to 4.5 cm (1.75 inches). The muscle spindles were again working and stopping the muscles, principally the ones in their necks, from over-contracting.

By using our bodies in the way that they were designed to be used, we can gain benefits that we may not have expected as well as feeling fitter, healthier and taller. For decades most people who practise the Alexander Technique have reported feeling taller – it can now be scientifically measured and proved that it actually happens.

Getting out of the car

The 'levering' that we talked about when standing up is widespread; you only have to watch people getting out of cars. They open the door and grip the edge of the windscreen or the steering wheel to lever

EXERCISE

Use this technique to get out of a car. Open the door of the car, swivel slightly so that your legs are out and then fall upright (see Figure 3.6). Try it and see if it's not easier. You'll be using gravity to work for you rather than against you. The levering is trying to defeat gravity, while the falling is using the weight of your head as a pivot around which the rest of your body weight swivels, until it has reached the upright position.

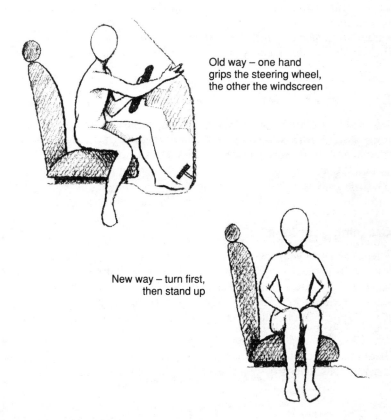

Old way – one hand grips the steering wheel, the other the windscreen

New way – turn first, then stand up

Figure 3.6 Getting out of the Car

themselves upright. A couple of decades of doing that and we have lost most of the strength and use of our involuntary muscles.

Confusing your brain

We have seen how the two different types of muscles work. As you go through your day it will be a useful exercise for you to try to see if you use the wrong sort of muscles for various activities. Remember, keeping your feet flat on the floor gives your body a good indication of which type of muscle it is supposed to be activating. However, there are several ways of confusing the system. If you sit with both feet flat on the floor, the message being relayed to your brain is that you are a standing up person and it will therefore switch on the postural, or involuntary, muscles and you can sit without getting tired for a long while.

Lying down people

If you then lift your feet up the message being delivered is that you are a lying down person and the brain will switch off the postural muscle and, if you are going to continue to sit upright, you will need to use the activity, or voluntary, muscles for support. The result of which is that you will get tired quickly. But what if you cross your legs? This is where you can confuse your brain dramatically.

Crossing your legs

When you cross your legs, the signals being delivered go haywire and the postural muscles along one side of the body will be switched on, while the muscles on the other side will be switched off. You will then invariably find yourself holding on to something, or propping yourself up in some way. You will sag to one side and need support (see Figure 3.7).

Moral superiority

Again remember there is no right or wrong way about anything we have discussed. You don't have to sit upright, you can cross your legs when you sit down, you can sag as much as you like. The Alexander Technique is about choice not rules. And it is not about judgement.

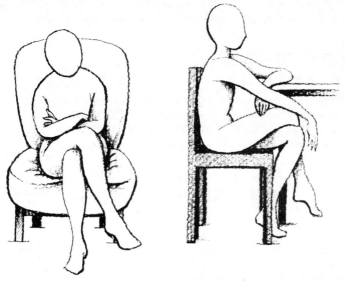

We have to use our arms to hold ourselves upright

Figure 3.7 Someone sitting with legs crossed

You may look at someone and think he or she is sitting badly, but it's up to that person and there is no moral superiority in standing 'better'. If it works for you do it, but do it quietly. You may find the Alexander Technique can produce the desired effect if you practise it yourself – telling other people that they need it or that they are standing badly can put them off ever wanting to learn about it. If it works for you that's great – let others wonder about your new graceful way of moving or increased health and vitality. If they want to know your secret they'll ask, and you can tell them, but meanwhile just concentrate on yourself.

The three ways of doing

There are only three ways of doing anything:

1 the way you would do it without thinking
2 the way you would do it if you were thinking
3 the way it's designed to be done.

Alexander said that the more you try to do it the right way, the more wrong you'll go. As soon as we have a concept of right or wrong we are liable to let that concept dictate to us the way we will stand – and it will be wrong (see Figure 3.8). It might not be the way we stand that is wrong but the concept most certainly will be. Because of the way we are brought up we have a concept of what is right and wrong that is based on false information supplied to us by others who knew no better themselves. While we hang on to our ideas of right and wrong we will always get it wrong. When we let go of our concepts we're in with a chance. We have to look at 'doing' in a fresh way.

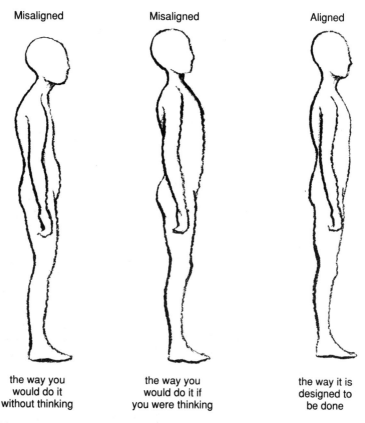

Misaligned	Misaligned	Aligned
the way you would do it without thinking	the way you would do it if you were thinking	the way it is designed to be done

Figure 3.8   The three ways of doing (standing)

—————— **The four stages of doing** ——————

The Alexander Technique aims to take you from Stage 1 of doing to Stage 4 of doing. Stage 1 is easy – you're doing it now. Stage 4 is easy – you were doing it when you were very young. It's the two stages in between that cause us problems. The four stages are:

- **Stage 1: Unconscious inefficiency** – this is the stage you're at – you don't do as you were designed to do;
- **Stage 2: Conscious inefficiency** – this is the stage you're arriving at – you don't do as you were designed to do, but you are now aware of it and can see the difference;
- **Stage 3: Conscious efficiency** – this is where you begin to do as you were designed to do, but you have to think about it and it feels strange;
- **Stage 4: Unconscious efficiency** – this is where it all becomes second nature and you again move with the grace and lightness of a child. You move efficiently and don't have to think about it – and it feels 'right'.

So if we're born at Stage 4 how come we end up at Stage 1 and have to relearn everything?

Developing bad habits

As children we learn to walk by falling forwards. Watch any child learning and you will see that each step is a falling into the next step. Children sit on the floor, squat, run around constantly and generally behave quite naturally. Then they go to school and it all starts to go horribly wrong. All their natural instincts to keep moving have to be suppressed and they are told to 'sit still!'. They also have to sit in chairs and we've seen how unfortunate that is. Then they have to sit in badly designed chairs and use their voluntary muscles to support themselves. Once learnt, it begins to feel 'right' and we continue that way. If you spend six hours a day as a small child in school being forced to commit your body to unnatural and highly awkward postures it's no wonder you get to believe it must be right. After all, it's the grown-ups who make you do it and surely they must know what they're doing?

All the evidence points to children growing faster than their parents – today's children are taller than ever before. The chairs and desks, however, haven't changed at all.

Who designed this, then?

If I could change any one of the three problems – sitting, sitting for long periods, and the design of the chairs – it would be the design I would go for. Chairs are not designed to fit humans – they're designed for ease of manufacture.

If you look closely at the way human beings are designed and compare it to the way the chairs are designed there seems to be a fundamental discrepancy. Chairs are hard and angular, invariably the back and seat are at right angles. Humans are soft and rounded with variable angles. Our thighs, when sitting, are not in their most relaxed position if at right angles to our backs (see Figure 3.9). If they are allowed to slope a little they find their most comfortable location. It is

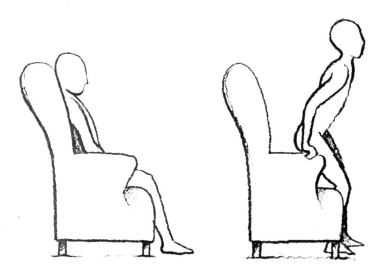

Figure 3.9 Conventional chair with someone trying to stand up

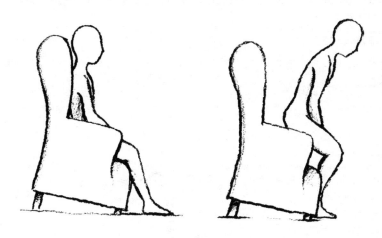

Figure 3.10 New chair with someone trying to stand up

also easy to stand up from a position where we are leaning slightly forwards – it makes us keep our feet flat on the floor which helps the internal sensors (see Figure 3.10). If we were to make the front legs of the chair a little shorter than the back legs it would improve things considerably. The position of the head would also be better placed to act as a counter balance when we stand up. The other problem with chairs is that they come in a uniform size while we don't.

Can you see what the problem is? I don't mean we should all go and chop a couple of centimetres off the front legs of our chairs, I just wanted you to be aware of the problem. You can always use a wedge-shaped cushion to give the same effect. You can make your own by cutting up blocks of foam or you can buy them from a suitable supplier (see 'Useful Information').

It gets worse

Once we've learnt to sit unnaturally and have the unnatural equipment – the chairs – it's only a matter of time before we sag. The teacher comes around and tells us to 'sit up straight'. This we do by arching our back and throwing our chest forwards (see Figure 3.11). It seems to do the trick because the teacher moves on to sort someone else out.

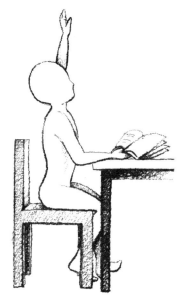

Figure 3.11   Small child sitting up straight

Maximum points for bad backs

As children we are told that an unnatural body posture earns us maximum points. So what do you think happens next? That's right, we adopt that unnatural posture whenever we want to impress, avoid trouble, receive praise, earn points, whatever. How many times were you told to stand up straight? Look back to Figure 3.11 and tell me how you learnt to sit up straight.

During our teen years slouching is a sign of indolence or rebellion, standing up straight is to do with conformity and thus goodness. And by the time we reach our twenties the conditioning has gone in hard and deep. We not only don't know how to place our bodies but we don't even know that we don't know.

Summary

Why should we ever have thought anything was wrong? Alexander was lucky in the sense that he had voice loss to point him in the direction of something being not right with his body. But us? It ain't broke – why should we do anything?

It may not be broke but I bet it's getting pretty close to it by now. Ever had backaches, stress, headache, muscular tension, tiredness, irritability, hypertension, breathing problems, insomnia, stiff neck, 'slipped disc', rheumatism, dietary problems, asthma?

A lot of common ailments can be directly attributed to using our bodies in a way that they were not designed to be used. The next chapter is about who can benefit from the Alexander Technique, but to summarise this chapter we learnt about:

- responses to stress
- letting go of excess tension
- the startle pattern
- the body's defence mechanisms
- internal sensors
- the two types of muscles
- the two systems of muscle nerves
- confusing the system
- the four stages of doing
- developing bad habits.

We will return to some of these in later chapters to consider them in more detail. Practise the exercises in this chapter and watch how others sit and stand. You could, while watching television, look out for the startle pattern. You can often see it on the news because people are being filmed in real situations. In plays or other entertainment it's often easy to spot when someone is 'acting' the startle pattern because they don't get it quite right. It's something quite hard to pretend to do and actors often get it wrong, but if you were to meet them in real life and tell them, *then* you'd see a perfect example of the startle pattern.

EXERCISE

See how much you use you hands and arms to support yourself
during your normal daily routine. We unconsciously pull ourselves
along and up quite a lot of the time. Try putting your hands behind
your neck, with your finger tips lightly resting on the back of your
neck, and then try: going up and down stairs; sitting down and
standing up; getting out of bed; getting out of a car. And please, no
accidents. You shouldn't need to hold on while doing any of the
above, but if you feel you'll hurt yourself then take care.

While you've got your finger tips on the back of your neck it's a useful exercise to feel what happens to your neck muscles as you walk
or run or whatever. Don't try to **do** anything at this stage – just
feel and be aware.

4
WHO CAN BENEFIT
FROM IT?

Everyone wants to be right, but no one stops to wonder if their idea of right is right.

F M Alexander

Frederick Alexander developed his technique originally for himself as a curative process to eliminate his constantly recurring problem of voice loss as an actor. Once he had diagnosed the cause of the problem, he went on to investigate all aspects of muscular control and tension elimination. However, his primary and overriding objective was to *cure* something that was wrong. Today the Alexander Technique is promoted mainly as a system of learning good body use and as a means of promoting health. But we mustn't lose sight of the fact that it was originally developed as a curative discipline – and it still works well as such today.

Case history

So, how did I get involved with the Alexander Technique? Well, when I was sixteen I played a lot of rugby and rode a lot of motor bikes. Eventually, by doing both, and one badly, I found I had seriously damaged the cartilage in my right knee. I went the round of doctors and hospitals, and it was recommended that I should have a major operation to remove and replace the cartilage. The surgeon told me there was an even chance that either I'd be fine or I wouldn't be able to walk. As I *could* walk, albeit painfully at times, I opted to do nothing.

For some twenty years I put up with a wonky knee. It meant I couldn't kneel properly, run properly or do much with it at all. It ached like blazes every winter when it got damp and it ached if I stood up for too long. It frequently let me down when I tried to run or ride a bike. All in all, it was a painful and limiting complaint – but I definitely wasn't going to have it operated on.

In my late thirties I happened to be visiting a friend who, unbeknownst to me, was training as an Alexander Technique teacher. He listened to me moaning about my knee as it was going through one of its painful phases. He looked at me and said that he could see little wrong except that the way I stood seemed awkward, as if I was holding my knee in a strange position. He suggested that, when I was standing upright, I should move my knee very slightly to a new position. It felt strange and unnatural, although I know now it was actually the 'correct' position for my knee to be in. I couldn't see how something so small and simple could make any difference. But it did.

Within a few months I had taken up a martial art, an activity I had thought closed to me forever. The pain in my knee disappeared as did the aches. I could run with it, kneel on it, and in general, do what anyone else could. I was naturally curious about this Technique, so I went for Alexander lessons. I quickly became a devotee, learnt all I could and even taught introductory classes myself for a while.

Today, I spend long periods in front of a computer screen and, as a writer, could be prone to stiff shoulders, aching muscles and a bad back. But I practise what I was taught and it keeps me supple and free of tension.

Moving after surgery

The real test came in the early 1990s when I was rushed to hospital one night with appendicitis. I was delirious and knew nothing about it until I awoke in the morning with stitches, pain and a full bladder. I had to get out of bed, but whenever I tried to pull myself upright the pain was too intense. Then I remembered. I was using my stomach muscles instead of gravity – it was the wall of my stomach that had been opened to allow the surgeon access to my appendix.

As soon as I realised where I was going wrong it was easy. I rolled on to my side, swung my legs to the floor and, using my body weight as a pivot, was able to stand upright without effort.

Once standing it was a different matter. Every time I tried to take a step, I stiffened with pain. Then I had to remember to inhibit – to unlearn trying to do and stop doing. It was a bit like learning to walk all over again. I couldn't use any muscular tension but had to allow my head to fall forwards which propelled me into the next step, much as a baby learns to walk by falling into the next step. I wasn't walking quickly but I *was* walking. And yes, I made it in time.

A post-operative therapy?

Within three days I was home and healing quickly. But I did notice while I was in hospital that other patients were having the same problems I'd had and realised that the Alexander Technique could be most beneficial as a post-operative therapy to get people moving again as quickly as possible. The quicker we start to move again after surgery the less risk there is of infection setting in.

———— Suitable candidates ————

So who can learn the Alexander Technique? Basically, anyone. You don't even have to be convinced that it will do anything for you – I certainly wasn't to begin with. In fact, I didn't know anything about it, not even what it was called. I just knew it worked. You may come to it because you have heard about it and are just interested, or you may have a major problem that has so far resisted all attempts by orthodox methods to be remedied, or you may even be sceptical. Whatever, your motivation, it is worth learning – it works.

Combining lessons

I assume you are interested or you wouldn't have got this far with this book. Learning it yourself works well but if you have a particular problem, like backache, then it's probably best if you combine self-teaching with a course of individual lessons. There's nothing quite like having an Alexander teacher pay you all the time and attention as well as helping you to correct things that have been wrong for a long time and you have not been able to resolve before. It's a nice feeling. Sometimes it's useful to have a refresher lesson just to check that you've still got the simplicity behind the Technique correct. It's so easy to add on and complicate things without even really trying. It may also be useful to have the odd lesson after reading a book such as this one. After all, what I write and what you read may turn out to be two different things. It's always useful just to check that we've both got it right. You could even attend one of the regular workshops on the Alexander Technique that take place (see 'Useful Information' for further details).

—— Suitable cases for treatment ——

The Society of Teachers of the Alexander Technique (STAT) says that the Alexander Technique 'addresses the fundamental causes of many cases of back pain, neck and shoulder tension, breathing disorders, stress-related illnesses and general fatigue where misuse and a loss of poise are contributory factors'. Many teachers have found that it is beneficial in treating a wide range of ailments – often these 'clear up' as a side effect or bonus. These ailments include:

- muscle fatigue
- migraine
- depression
- high blood pressure
- hypertension
- stress-related disorders including ulcers, eating disorders and digestion problems
- circulatory problems
- backache problems
- respiratory problems
- speech defects.

There are many other problems, complaints and disorders that people have that can benefit from the Alexander Technique. There's no need to list detailed case histories here – we are all different and what affects someone with a particular complaint may not affect others in the same way. How are we supposed to be? Fit, active and healthy. If not, then let's try to change it.

—— Freeing ourselves from illness ——

Practising the Alexander Technique allows us to harmonise our bodies, minds and emotions. Once we have this harmony, we are more able to free ourselves from illness. There is an old Chinese saying: 'In the West when something happens they ask what they can do about it – here in the East we ask what caused it.' The Alexander Technique is a way of looking at what causes our bodies to malfunction. Invariably, it's because we didn't know how they were supposed to function in the first place. Once we learn how we are supposed to be, we can practise it.

EXERCISE

Quick exercise to see how body shape can affect respiratory problems.

1 Scrunch yourself up as tight and as tense as you can, pull your head down into your body and shorten and tense your neck, clench your fists with your arms pressed tightly across your chest. Now take the deepest breath you can and see how long you can hold it. Let it out and say 'ahhh' as you do so.

2 Now let go of all that tension, allow your body to lengthen and widen, head up and out, arms loosely by your side, smile. Now take the deepest breath you can and hold it. Let it out and say 'ahhh' as you do so.

3 Compare the two results. In 1 the deep breath is nowhere as deep as in 2, and the time you can hold that deep breath is much shorter. Also, in 2 the 'ahhh' is deeper, richer, more resonate that in 1. How can you breath properly if you're tense and scrunched up?

Your approach

Some Alexander Technique teachers report quite staggering results with arthritis, rheumatism and asthma, often as an unlooked for bonus. If you suffer from any of these conditions and they have not responded to orthodox treatments, or you wish to check out a more natural method, then seeing a qualified Alexander teacher can do you no harm. Learning the Technique can only improve your basic body poise and that is something we can all benefit from. Expecting dramatic results is probably not the best way to approach the Alexander Technique – it's too subtle for that. It's best to adopt a 'try it and see' approach. Then, when it works, you'll be delighted. But if the effects are relatively small, you will be more philosophical than disappointed.

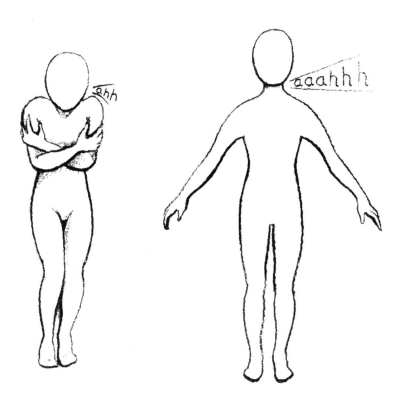

Figure 4.1 A quick exercise

Healthy teeth

The benefits of the Technique can have far reaching effects that we wouldn't even think of. If I told you that the health of my teeth has improved, you'd probably think I was imagining it. However, it's a fact that was pointed out to me by my dentist – and she didn't even know I was doing (or not doing) anything. Quite simply, I had learnt to question the way I did *everything* and I was experimenting with trying to change my habits. I noticed that I was always brushing my teeth by leaning on the basin with my left arm, bending over, tensing up, and twisting slightly to the right while I brushed vigorously with the toothbrush in my right hand. The only way I could stop myself hanging on with my left arm, a totally unproductive exercise, was to swop hands. I tried brushing my teeth holding the brush first in one hand and then the other. It felt very strange so I knew I was on to something. Anyway you know the rest. Using a different hand to hold the toothbrush meant I was cleaning the back teeth on the lower right side of my mouth better than they had ever been cleaned before: less decay and thus fewer fillings. An unexpected bonus indeed.

Improving performance

Alexander, being an actor, naturally promoted his new discoveries amongst fellow entertainers. Musicians latched on pretty quickly, followed by athletes and dancers. Today, anyone who uses their body in complicated habitual manoeuvres can benefit, and that includes just about all of us. Learning how to do what we do with a new poised posture can only be helpful.

Wasting energy

If every time we move we expend valuable energy it makes sense to move with minimum effort – wasting energy is not only exhausting, but also unproductive. If this sounds a little serious you may like to look at it another way: all the energy you later save can be used for activities you really like. Why waste energy sitting down and standing up when you could save it and spend it later doing something much more interesting?

The three types of candidates

Basically, I see people who want to learn the Technique as being one of three types:

- people who want to learn it in the hope it will alleviate a specific condition or complaint
- people who want to learn it to help improve a particular thing they do with their bodies, like dancers or musicians
- people who want to learn it for general interest.

Occasionally you do get someone who doesn't fit into any of these categories. At one Introductory Workshop I was running I asked all the people there why they were attending. Everyone fitted into one of the three categories except one woman who was strangely reluctant to reveal why she was there. With a little gentle probing I got to the real reason, and it's nothing horrendous. It was merely that she was a journalist from a national newspaper, who'd been sent along to find out what it was all about. She wrote her article and still practises regularly.

At another workshop, again everyone fitted into the three categories except one woman. Why was she there? Quite simple, she explained, the Alexander Technique was the only therapy she hadn't yet done. A therapy collector.

—— # End gainers and A types ——

We talked earlier about end gaining and you may already know about A and B types. In case you don't, here's a brief summary:

- **A Types** – impatient, aggressive, ambitious, hurrying, rushed, quick, stressed, demanding, difficult, loud, creative, leading, rousing, dynamic, confident, decisive;
- **B Types** – patient, defensive, relaxed, considerate, cautious, careful, following, receptive, caring, nervous, questioning, indecisive, quiet, philosophical, thorough.

Which are you?

I'm sure you can add many more attributes to both lists. Which type are you? Probably a good mixture of both, but most of us want to be more B than A. We all know that B types live longer, suffer fewer heart problems, less stress, fewer frustrations and setbacks, because they think things through more, have a calmer outlook, are more laid back and are generally nicer people. But A types can have more fun living on the edge, more excitement, are better at solving (and probably causing) problems, exploring, discovering, creating and leading. I have no desire to give up my A-ness, I just want to be less end gaining about it. The Alexander Technique allows us to be ourselves without having to change our basic personality (we can if we want – it's all to do with choice). Sometimes we need A types around and sometimes B types. I wouldn't like to be facing danger with a B – that's the time you need an A.

B types have their downside, too. They appear to be more prone to carcinogens, more prone to neurosis and mental disorders, less likely to achieve or 'reach the top', more prone to worry and sleep disorders, more prone to dietary disorders and respiratory problems.

Living with the two types

We are what we are, there's no better or worse. I have two sons, one an A and the other a B. I tend to think of them as Mr Bouncy and Mr Book. There is no way I love either more or less. Each is different and equally wonderful. They will both go through life encountering their own set of problems and solving them in the way they are uniquely equipped to do. Mr Bouncy will rush at everything and keep doing so until the problem is resolved. Mr Book will think long and hard, and eventually the problem will go away of its own accord. Each way creates it's own problems and each way works – for them. (I also have a daughter, but she's an O type – oh, dad, I need more money; oh dad, I haven't got enough clothes; oh dad, I need a lift!)

Changes to your basic personality

If you think I've gone on a lot about this, it's because the Alexander Technique requires you to make no changes to your basic personality. It's fine to be who you are: you'll just be moving more gracefully being you. You don't have to give up anything except your tension. You don't have to believe any philosophy, you just have to try it. If it works, do it; if it doesn't, don't. You don't have to believe anything, it's all subject to testing and results. A types will ask, 'What can this do for me?', B types will want to know, 'How will it make me feel?'

How A types will benefit

A types will benefit because they, by becoming more relaxed and expending less energy, can get more done. They will be able to move faster, be less clumsy and suffer fewer accidents. They will be able to pace themselves better and not have to recover quite so often.

How B types will benefit

B types will benefit because they will feel fitter and healthier and more in harmony. They will increase their understanding of themselves, have a valuable insight to share with their friends and families, and be more dynamic because of their increased energy levels. They will be more confident, poised and capable.

How to tell if others are A or B

If you're still wondering which you are, A or B, then you're probably a B. And if you want to know what someone else is, try not finishing a sentence when you're talking to them. A types will finish it for you, B types will allow you the space to finish it, sometimes even making little encouraging noises to help you.

———— Taking responsibility ————

There is a tendency in the West to blame our problems on others: we can't get on because we're being held back; if only so and so was nicer to us we'd be happier; if only you loved me more my life would be better; it's all your fault I'm the way I am. Once you take responsibility for your body you take responsibility for your outlook. Alexander knew full well the vital connection between body poise and emotional well-being. It's no good blaming everyone for the shape we're in. No amount of blaming will alter it one tiny bit. Even if you could gather all your teachers together and tell them off and they were to all confess their faults and apologise to you, you would get not one jot better. You're who you are now, and only you can affect change. By not blaming, and instead taking responsibility for who and how we are, we can make positive changes. Once we make those changes our outlook improves: we are already improving because we are making changes. It's a non-vicious circle, a benign upward spiral if you like.

Treating depression

The more we blame, the less we do about it. I have seen some very dramatic improvements in people suffering severe depression when they've been taught the Alexander Technique.

EXERCISE

Just in case you need a little proof, try the following. First adopt the classic 'depressed' body shape – allow your shoulders to hunch, drop your head, frown and pull your mouth down at the corners, tense your whole body inwardly as if expecting a blow, and say out loud 'I feel absolutely miserable'. Now you know why it's called *depression* – you have just physically depressed your entire body.

Now let all that tension go and adopt the 'happy' posture – head up, smile, open body shape, relaxed, confident, and say out loud 'I feel fantastic!'.

Now try adopting the depressed posture and say out loud 'I feel fantastic!'
Now adopt the happy posture and say 'I feel absolutely miserable.' See what happens. When we physically depress ourselves we feel depressed. When we physically open up, so do our feelings. It's almost impossible to feel happy if our bodies are shut down, and it's a whole lot easier to feel less depressed if we're not physically depressed.

Simple test

So you may be asking if *you* can benefit. Simple test – stop reading and go and find a full-length mirror. Take all your clothes off and have a look at yourself sideways. If there's anything in your posture that you're not happy about, you can change it. Yes, you can benefit.

What makes the Alexander Technique so different?

The Alexander Technique is not therapy or a discipline. I like to think of it as an operating system. An analogy I use is that it's a bit like having a computer. You have to have *software* (your programs, such as a word processing package or some games to play) and you have to have some *hardware* (your screen, keyboard, printer and CPU – the big box that contains the Central Processing Unit that sits on your desk), and you have to have an *operating system* (usually called something like MS-DOS; the system that tells your computer how to set itself up, which language to speak, what to do when you turn it on and how to load and use the software. Well, therapies or disciplines or whatever we do are the software, your body is the hardware and the Alexander Technique is the operating system. The one we normally have is built out of bits at random, bits left over from childhood, school, wherever. By learning a new operating system we link the hardware and software together to work efficiently. In normal use you don't see the operating system, and so it is with the Alexander Technique. Once installed it should not be visible.

How the Technique fits in with other disciplines

You can use the principles of the Alexander Technique to improve any other activity you do. A question often asked is, 'Which should I learn, the Alexander Technique or something like Tai Ch'i or yoga or aerobics?' Well, you can use the principles of the Alexander Technique when you're learning, say, Tai Ch'i and you'll find them helpful and they definitely add something. I'm not sure it works the other way round. I would suggest that the Alexander Technique is something you learn first then you can learn any of the others and do them well. If you learn the others first you may well be doing them in a way that isn't completely efficient right from the start. If you already practise another discipline try to apply some of the principles you're leaning here and see if it changes anything.

Summary

It's taken a lot to answer the question posed by this chapter. I think the quickest answer to the question 'Who can benefit from it?' is: you, me, anyone, everyone, all of us.

And it's not just something we learn, get good at and then think we've done it. Alexander took ten years developing it, taught it for over fifty years, and it was said that he did his best work in the last five years of his life. He was still developing it to the very end.

Once you've learnt the Technique you can apply it to new situations as they occur, change and adapt it as you change and adapt in your life, constantly monitor it as you put it into practice, use it to refresh yourself whenever you feel you're going back into old habits, and find new ways to incorporate it into your daily life. It's an operating system: once learnt it just sits in the background helping you to operate efficiently.

5

HOW IS IT DONE WITH GUIDANCE?

When anything is pointed out our only idea is to go from wrong to right, in spite of the fact that it has taken us years to get wrong: we try to get right in a moment.

F M Alexander

Frederick Alexander learnt and knew his Technique better than anyone else has ever done, yet he never had a single lesson in his life. So how important are lessons? If you ask the Society of Teachers of the Alexander Technique (STAT) they will say that 'you learn to appreciate the practical implications of thought and its effort on muscle activity. A teacher's hands encourage a specific quality of muscle tone. This, together with words of instruction, helps to release inappropriate tension and allows the body to become better aligned and balanced.' They advocate lessons as being very important.

Watching yourself

I believe that you can, like Alexander himself, learn a great deal from watching yourself. Probably the best approach is to learn all you can from books so that you have a thorough grounding in the principles, and then have some lessons to make sure you're putting it all into practice as efficiently as possible. STAT advises a course of a minimum of twenty lessons for 'continuing self-improvement' and says 'a few lessons can make a difference'. I've found that lessons help me correct specific faults and learning from books has given me an understanding of how it works, but the most I've learnt has certainly been from self-observation. Lessons work well during the actual lesson. But if you're anything like me you'll forget everything you were shown the minute you walk out of the treatment room. I can do anything with perfectly relaxed poise when I want to demonstrate or impress: it's much more difficult when I have to apply it all unconsciously, or when I encounter new situations like waking up in hospital.

What does it cost?

STAT advises that lessons should cost (at the time of writing this book) between £14 and £25 which means you could be paying around £500 for your recommended *minimum* of twenty lessons. However, it may be that medical insurance from such major providers as BUPA and WPA often covers the cost of lessons when they have been recommended by a consultant as part of a treatment plan. In some cases the NHS funds lessons.

A typical lesson

Let's run through exactly what happens when you go for your individual lesson. Let's suppose you have chosen a qualified teacher (details in 'Useful Information'), made your first appointment and arrived at their place of teaching. You don't have to wear anything special, although loose, light clothing like a track suit is suggested as anything tight and heavy restricts not only your movements, but also your teacher's observations of you and how you move. You will not need to remove any clothing for the lesson. The lessons last about thirty to forty-five minutes and should be relaxing and enjoyable. There's no-one else there apart from your teacher, so don't worry about making a fool of yourself, or competing or performing. You won't be asked to do anything difficult.

You may well be asked why you have decided to come for lessons, so it's good to be clear in your own mind beforehand.

Disturbing questions?

The teacher will not ask you any probing or disturbing questions about your childhood, sex life of lifestyle, so you don't have to worry about revealing anything you may be embarrassed about, or reluctant to discuss. You may be asked in a general way what you do and if you're a family person. That's partly so that the teacher can get an idea of what sort of person you are and what sort of routine you might have. It's more likely to be general conversation designed to relax you and put you at ease. The teacher doesn't need to know anything about you, except how you move. Anything else you choose to tell your teacher is entirely up to you, it can be as much or as little as you want.

Medical history and medication

I would suggest that if you have any physical disability or complaint you should tell your teacher in advance. You may have a particular medical history that precludes you from having lessons. If you're not sure, discuss it with your teacher and/or your doctor. And if you are receiving any medication you should check with both your teacher and your doctor that having lessons will in no way interfere with your treatment.

Ask any questions you want to – they should be answered easily and openly.

Your first lesson

The first few minutes of your first lesson will probably be spent chatting. This helps put you at your ease and lets you and your teacher get to know each other. Most teachers will then ask you to stand up or sit down while they place their hands gently on your neck. This is so they can feel how tense you are, how you perform simple movements and so that you get used to them touching you. Some people find it quite emotionally uncomfortable to have a stranger touch them, even in this sort of a way.

Your teacher may well give you a short introductory talk about what the Alexander Technique is – or rather isn't. So many people go to their first lesson full of concepts of how it's about posture and standing up straight. Teachers often say that it takes longer to re-educate people than to educate them in the principles of the Alexander Technique.

Your teacher may ask you to carry out some simple movements like sitting down and standing up, lying down and getting up. They will probably ask you to do these several times. The first few times you will be conscious of them watching you, you may even try to do them 'properly', but eventually you relax, forget that the teacher is there and just do them in the same old way you would at home. Then your teacher can see how you really move. Your teacher may ask about any accidents or injuries you've had during your life. You've probably forgotten most of them, so it may be helpful if you spend some time before the lesson making a note of them.

What shape are you in?

You may be asked to walk up and down a few times so the teacher can see how you do it, and to stand with your back against a wall. This is so that the teacher can see how your back is shaped. All in all, you'll be thoroughly observed, and won't notice at all.

The semi-supine position

Your teacher may ask you to lie in the *semi-supine position*. We will go into this in greater depth in Chapter 6, but basically you lie on the floor on your back with your knees bent and some hard books under your head (see Figure 5.1). This position, when adopted properly encourages your back to lengthen and widen as well as correcting your head–neck relationship. You may well be given this position to practise for about fifteen minutes twice a day as 'homework' between lessons.

While you are lying in the semi-supine position, your teacher may place your arms, head and legs in a slightly different position from the one you are in. They're straightening you out. It may feel odd or awkward but you can trust them. Standing above you they can see much more clearly how straight you're lying. They're also trained to do this. If they move you, go with the movement. Don't resist.

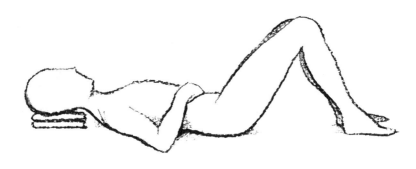

Figure 5.1   Semi-supine position

Give them the weight. What this means is that if you are resisting, your teacher may ask you to 'give me the weight'. You should go completely limp. Be like a dead thing: no resistance, no tension, no thought of where you're supposed to be placing your body. Let your teacher do it; they're trained, qualified and being paid to do it. You just relax and enjoy the experience of realising that you haven't got a clue what you 'should' be doing, what you 'think' you should be doing, or even whether you should be doing anything at all.

Little monkeys

You may well be shown the classic *monkey* stance, or *position of mechanical advantage* to give it its technical name. This again will be explained fully in Chapter 6. Essentially, you'll be shown how to stand bending slightly from the hips and with your knees also slightly

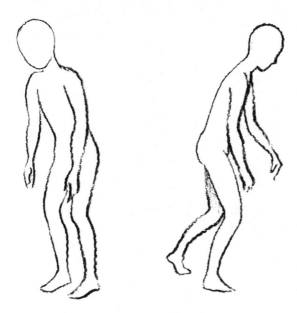

Figure 5.2 Monkey position

bent (see Figure 5.2). This teaches you about the most efficient head–neck–back relationship.

Hands on

Your teacher may well stand you up and sit you down several times while keeping one hand on the back of your neck and the other on the top of your head (see Figure 5.3). As you stand up and sit down your teacher will make minute adjustments to the position of your head and neck. During a course of lessons the 'feel' of where your head is supposed to be becomes more natural, although at first it will feel quite strange.

Ahhh

If your teacher asks you to breathe out while making an 'ahhh' sound, this isn't to check your tonsils or vocal chords. It's to get you to let

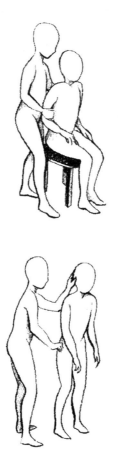

Figure 5.3 Teacher with hands on

your ribcage expand. This allows the back to lengthen and widen. The 'ahhh' sound also teaches you what a loose jaw feels like, and a loose jaw is a relaxed jaw. Many people hold their jaw extremely rigid. Making the 'ahhh' sound as you breath out relaxes most of your face as well. As you make the sound you are encouraged to smile – more relaxation. The 'ahhh' is not spoken with the vocal chords, but rather the sound of the breath coming out of your mouth as you release all the tension you are holding.

Other practices

You may be asked to kneel, crawl, squat, and even run. It all depends on individual teachers and how they think you need directing and correcting. You may even be asked to adopt the Muslim prayer position (see Figure 5.4). No, not to pray, but so you can feel what's happening to your back.

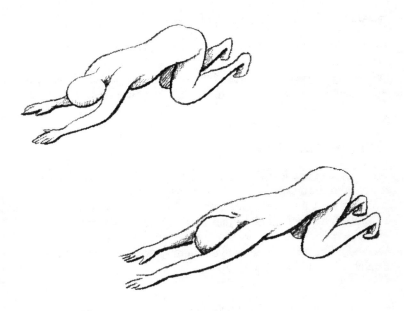

Figure 5.4   Muslim prayer position

Different strokes for different folks

Individual teachers may have other exercises and positions I haven't mentioned here. Your lesson will be tailored to suit you and, as such, may be very different from what anyone else has or doesn't have. There's no point comparing with anyone else. There's not a lot of point competing either. The only way of monitoring your progress is by how you feel.

Homework

You may be given exercises to practise at home in between lessons. You will be given directions – conscious projections – to say to yourself as you go about your daily tasks. These will probably be: let the neck be free; let the head go forwards and up; allow the back to lengthen and widen.

Subsequent lessons

Your follow-up lessons will usually be much the same as the first lesson. You may find you think you've got the Technique just right only to keep being corrected every time you go for a lesson. Then, when you're convinced you've got it wrong, you're teacher will tell you that you've got it right.

Will I be able to do it?

Yes. It's much like learning to drive a car. You have a lot to remember at first and it all takes some getting used to. Then, when you're least expecting it, it falls into place and you're driving. Looking back I bet it's quite hard to remember just how difficult it was when you first learnt to drive, but now you don't even think about it. Learning the Alexander Technique is the same. There's a lot that's new at first, but it quickly becomes second nature.

The teachers

Alexander teachers are ordinary people, like you and me, who have decided to make being a teacher of the Alexander Technique their profession. They do it for a living. It's not a hobby or a calling. It's their profession. And as such you should treat it in the same way you would treat a visit to your doctor, dentist, osteopath or whoever. Keep your appointments, arrive on time, pay their fees on time and treat them in a professional manner. That also means that they are working for you. If you are unhappy or have a complaint then tell them, and expect them to accommodate your needs. If you continue to be unhappy with the service provided then change your teacher. You don't have to stick with a teacher you don't particularly get on with, either. They, like us, are all different. You may find one you really relate to straight away. You may find you need to try several before making your final choice. Listen to other people's recommendations. Go to introductory courses. Get the list of qualified teachers from STAT (see 'Useful Information'). Shop around until you're satisfied, and then go for it. The Alexander Technique teaches natural body poise: it's not a therapy or a religion or a cult or a 'new age' manipulation process. It's a professional learning method, a science, if you like, taught by teachers who belong to an extremely professional governing body. These professional teachers have to be approved by the Society.

Understanding artists

Jane Foulkes, in her book *Complementary Medicine Careers Handbook*, says:

> *Ideally, the person who will make a good Alexander Teacher will combine an artistic interest in physical self-expression with a scientific interest in anatomy, physiology and psychology. If you are going to help performing artists it is especially helpful if you have experience of their particular art, so that you can quickly come to an understanding of its demands on the body and mind as well as the emotions.*

How do you get approved?

To qualify as a member of STAT teachers have to complete a three-year training course and reach a standard that the Society considers competent. The course is full time and the teachers have to abide by a strict, published code of ethics. It costs teachers around £9000 to complete the course so they have to be dedicated. They are expected to have completed a full course of Alexander Technique lessons themselves before they can enrol as trainee teachers.

Grants

You may be able to get a discretionary grant to pay for course fees from your local authority, especially where the candidate has the backing of a relevant respected local body or national organisation.

Obviously it's dependent on the amounts of money available at any one time, and on the options of the grants committee.

Who's suitable?

According to STAT, candidates 'must have good health, character and education and (normally) be aged between the ages of 18 and 35. Since Alexander teachers are often called upon to work with people of widely differing ages, needs and interests, almost any form of previous training and experience can be an advantage, but none is essential.'

Course content

During their three-year course, students work in small groups of five or fewer with their course instructor. Their work is mainly of a practical nature but time is given for lectures and discussions on basic anatomy, physiology, the Technique itself, practical demonstrations and other related topics.

The students begin by practising on each other and may be allowed access, in their final year, to members of the public. They will be monitored throughout their course in their own use and understanding of the Alexander Technique. By the time they get to you they know their subject well.

Workshops and introductory groups

As more and more people get to hear about the Alexander Technique there has been an increased demand for STAT to organise some way of explaining what it is about to interested people. They arrange for qualified teachers to demonstrate and explain the Technique at introductory workshops and it may be useful for you to attend one. You don't have to pay for a course of lessons, but you do get to see the Technique being demonstrated in a practical way. These workshops are usually one-day introductory courses, and they take place in all sorts of places throughout the world. Please see 'Useful Information' for details of addresses of STAT worldwide. You can contact them in your country and they will give you all the information you require regarding where and when workshops are scheduled. For the United Kingdom you need to contact their London headquarters. The introductory workshops will cost you anything from nothing to £30 a day to attend and some teachers will even give a free half-hour introductory lesson.

You can also learn the Alexander Technique under the auspices of the Local Education Authority in some area. You need to check with your town hall or library to see if workshops or classes are available in your area.

How widespread is the Alexander Technique?

To give you some idea, there are over 500 teaching members of STAT in the United Kingdom alone. There are teachers in most, if not all, European countries as well as Israel, Africa, the United States and Australia. Worldwide there are over 1200 members, and STAT is the internationally recognised governing body. There is even an Alexander Trust, which is a registered charity, set up in 1990 to advance the education of the public and to promote research and study into all aspects of the Technique.

There is a STAT bookshop (address in 'Useful Information') which sells books on the subject as well as tapes, videos, newsletters and even posters of Alexander himself.

Summary

Have lessons if you need to correct a particular fault or to check you are using the Technique properly. Some people keep their lessons going on a regular basis for years. Others have one or two and then find they have learnt enough to help them. It's up to you to decide what you need. Have lessons only from a qualified STAT approved teacher if you feel you want lessons, but remember Alexander himself never had a single lesson in his life. Anyway, that's enough about lessons – it's time you learnt more about how to do it for yourself.

6

HOW TO DO IT FOR YOURSELF

When you get what you 'feel' is the right position and you have imperfect co-ordination, you are only getting a position which fits with your defective co-ordination.

F M Alexander

- A system of postural re-education and good body use;
- General improvement in the use of the body from which correction of individual detailed faults will follow;
- A means for changing stereotyped response patterns by the inhibition of certain postural sets;
- A method for expanding consciousness to take in inhibition as well as excitation and thus obtaining a better integration of the reflex and voluntary elements in a response pattern;
- A method of posture training;
- A technique by which mind and body are harmonised;
- Learning to move your joints and muscles correctly;
- A series of physical movements designed to correct bad posture and bring the body back into alignment, thus helping it to function efficiently, as nature intended.

These are all definitions of the Alexander Technique from teachers, authors and psychologists. It's interesting to look at what Alexander himself had to say when asked to sum it up. He said: 'How can you name something which is so comprehensive. If you do what I did, you'll be able to do what I do.' And what he did was to consciously examine every movement he made and then analyse why and how. Once he was aware of the movement, he learnt to *inhibit* to prevent the old habits controlling the movements and then to substitute new controls – *conscious projections* – to replace the habits, and then to move using *primary control* – allowing his head and neck to be free and properly aligned. Those essentially are the three stages of the Alexander Technique. Now we have to learn how to put it all into practice.

Misconceptions

Before we begin, I would like to clear up a few popular misconceptions that arise around any teaching of the technique:

- **Inhibitions** – These are nothing to do with the Freudian concept of suppressed or repressed emotions. Inhibitions, in Alexander terminology, means stopping and thinking before making a movement to give yourself a chance to change your mind and not continue with the movement, or to continue, or to do something else. The inhibition is done *before* any movement has taken place. It's a tiny pause before you move while you consider the value of the movement;

- **Conscious projection** – This is not a meaningless mantra to be repeated to dull or empty the mind. It is a *conscious* instruction to yourself *before* you make a movement and *while* you are making it. The conscious projection is: *let the neck be free, let the head go forwards and up, allow the back to lengthen and widen.* Conscious projection is a thought; it is not a movement of any sort, whatsoever. You think it, you don't *do* it. You are *letting* and *allowing.* This is not movement, it is permission;

- **Primary control** – The head should be directed up and forwards. First: up is *not* a place, it is a direction. It is the direction that the top of the spine happens to be pointing in. When you're sitting or standing, then *up* is towards the ceiling, but if you are lying down then *up* is towards the head of the bed. And if you were crawling, *up* would be towards the wall in front of you. Second: directing the head *forwards* does not mean you thrust it forwards. Forwards, again, is a direction. You tilt your head, where it balances on top of the spine (between the ears, not the top of the neck), until it is directed forwards.

Please read and re-read these three points until they are fully and instinctively understood. They are probably the most important aspect of learning the Technique. We can go no further until they are second nature. However, as Alexander said, 'we can throw away the habits of a lifetime in a few minutes if we use our brains'.

Are you aligned?

EXERCISE

After all these years of not making proper *use* of yourself, you may be *out of alignment*. If you were having lessons it would be one of the first things your teacher would look for. So how do you know whether you're out of alignment? Try this simple exercise. Find yourself an area of blank wall. You should be wearing light clothes, or no clothing on at all, and be barefoot. Stand with your back to the wall and position your feet so that they are 45 cm (18 inches) apart with your heels 5 cm (2 inches) out from the wall. I suggest that you actually measure and mark on the floor those two measurements. It's easy to get them wrong when you're looking down at your feet from above.

At first, don't touch the wall at all. Then relax and let yourself lean gently back against the wall. If you are well aligned your shoulder blades and buttocks will touch the wall all at the same time. These are your *three points of reference* (see Figure 6.1).

If one shoulder blade touches before another, then you are slightly twisted or *one-sided*. If your buttocks touch first, you are holding your pelvis too far back. If your shoulders touch first, you are holding your pelvis too far forwards.

Now you're leaning back, can you feel what is touching? I bet there's a big gap between your lower back and the wall.

Try this exercise every morning when you first get out of bed and again last thing at night before you collapse.

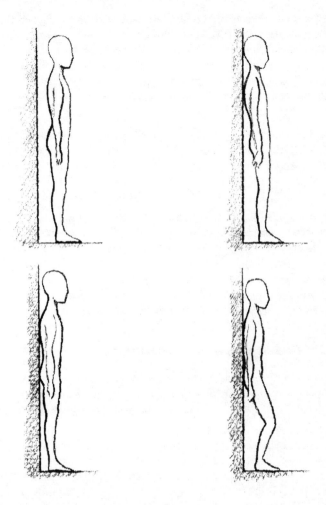

Figure 6.1 Leaning against a wall - 4 stages

Help! I'm out of alignment

First of all, don't panic. We're all out of alignment to some extent and we can put it right. If you find that there's that gap between your lower back and the wall, try bending your legs at the knees slightly until the gap disappears – you will have to slide down the wall a bit (see Figure 6.1). Let your arms hang loosely at your sides and don't *do* anything. Stay like this for a while. This is a useful exercise for correcting misalignments, but only if you actually do it. Gradually, over a period, you will find that you touch the wall at all three reference points at the same time and the gap will go. If you still touch one shoulder blade first, you are allowed to *un-twist* so that you are touching at all three points.

You may find that the feeling of standing with your back to the wall, without your knees bent, can be quite strange – it feels as if you are leaning backwards. However, I can guarantee you that you are standing more upright than you have for a long time. It's all to do with the centre of gravity. It's never where we think it is. More about that later.

If you are out of alignment you may find standing with your knees bent fairly uncomfortable to begin with. Persevere – it will get easier, I promise you. I suggest you try this a few times to get to know how you feel and then incorporate it into a routine of exercise to correct matters. You can use the time to remember the three vital points – inhibit, project, control. Do them as you stand there, do them as you lean backwards, do them as you correct your alignment.

How did I get out of alignment?

I don't know how *you* personally got out of alignment – we are all different and all end up the same place although we may arrive by different routes. There may, however, be a few things we all have in common.

Stand against the wall again, legs straight, and now lift your heels a couple of centimetres off the ground. What happens to your alignment? Try doing the exercise as before right from the start, but this time do it on tip-toe. What happens now? You'll probably find it quite hard to touch your buttocks against the wall without bending your knees or contorting your back. That's the effect you get everyday when you wear shoes with heels on them. Now can you explain why we wear shoes with heels? We don't need them, so what's it all about? I don't know the answer to any of these questions but you might like to think about them while you're standing against the wall. Why are all kitchen units a standard height when we're not? Why are most beds a standard height? Why are chairs, stairs and steps all a standard height? Why are train seats so uncomfortable? Why are the foot pedals in cars where they are?

EXERCISE

Stand with your back to the wall. While you're getting used to standing there for a while with all three reference points touching and your knees bent, I have a question for you. Where's your head, and why? It's not a trick question. You don't suddenly have to wonder if you've missed something. I never said where it *should* be. If you stand against the wall realigning yourself, your head will find its own place. You might like to try letting the back of your head touch the wall. What does that feel like? Comfortable? I think not. Ideally your head is in its best position a couple of inches out from the wall. If it's not don't worry; the *semi-supine* exercise later on will realign it. By the way, if you live with someone you may need to explain what you are doing. You may have a little fun poked at you. That's OK. The Alexander Technique can be fun. It doesn't all have to be terribly serious. You can always elicit the help of your partner. I do. Every now and again, just to check, I ask 'Where's my head?' The usual answer is 'I don't know, where did you leave it?' But after the jokes I'm usually told 'sticking forwards, hiding between your shoulders'. Yep, that's me. Knowing I'm round-shouldered and looking like a turtle is helpful, believe me. Because now I can do something about it. If I find myself slumped in front of the television I can do something about it if I want to. Now there's an interesting expression – *if I find myself*. It's as if someone put me there. I think not. Let's go back. When I choose to slump in front of the television I can do something about it. By altering my position I can regain my poise.

— The two parts of the Technique —

Any teaching of the Technique has to be divided into two parts; both have to be learnt and practised simultaneously. In a book we can progress only in a linear fashion so we have to work through the points separately.

What we are doing and the way we are doing it

First, we have to find out *what* we are doing and whether the *way* we are doing it is efficient and fits in with the body's design. And then we look at *how* what we are doing affects us. In other words find the habits, find how we do them and check what they are doing to us.

The best use of ourselves

Second, we have to find new ways of doing that make the best *use* of ourselves, doing efficiently and according to the best features of the body design. And stop the habits re-occurring. In other words, replace the habits, find new ways to do and then enjoy experiencing our new poise and gracefulness in movement.

Getting the hang of it?

OK, back against the wall, legs bent. When you're ready, and after *inhibiting, projecting* and *controlling*, walk away slowly from the wall for a few steps. What does it feel like? And no, you don't have to walk around like this all the time. Just take a few steps in this new position. It's not right or wrong – it's just new. You haven't walked around like this for a while, maybe not even in this lifetime, but a few million years ago humans were walking like this all the time. It's the missing step between walking on all fours and walking upright.

As you walk around for a few steps let all the tension go. I bet you'll be holding your chest stiffly. Let your arms hang loosely and make the 'ahhh' sound we did earlier. Lighten up and let it all go.

Now walk backwards to the wall and see which bit touches first. I bet it was the buttocks. Walk away and walk backwards. Which bit now? Again the buttocks. And it will be for quite a while. When you do the standing against the wall in the mornings and evenings, walk away like this and see how quickly you revert to your old walk, and why? There should be a nice in-between stage – in between this funny new walk and your funny old walk there is a stage of lightness and grace. As you pass through it see if you can feel it. By experiencing it a couple of times it will become familiar, and then in later exercises you may well know the feeling you will be aiming for.

—— Are you sitting comfortably? ——

EXERCISE

I want you to arrange three seating positions:

1 a standard hard-backed chair, like a kitchen chair
2 a couple of telephone directories on the floor to a height of about 15 cm (6 inches) – (or the distance between your finger tips and wrist)
3 nothing at all

I want you to sit first in the chair and notice where all the bits of you end up. How's your back? Your head? Your torso? Your legs and feet? These aren't trick questions – there's no right or wrong. Just have a look at yourself and see where you put everything.

Now sit cross-legged on the pile of directories. You can let your legs splay out in front of you with just your ankles crossed if it's more comfortable. Or you can raise your knees. Or splay your legs out completely. Again where is everything? How does it feel?

Now sit on the floor with nothing to support you. You can try to sit cross-legged or again splay your legs. How is everything this time?

Choosing our seating position

Now I want you to choose which of these three positions you would choose if you could choose only one to keep for the rest of your life. I don't know which you would choose, but I'd go for the pile of directories. It's a nice height. There's plenty of choice about where I can put my legs. It feels comfortable and natural. I can't slump and, most importantly, I can sit there for hours without getting uncomfortable. So why is my desk at a regulation height, forcing me to sit on a hard chair? It's off to Japan for me where they understand these things. The second sitting position is close to our natural sitting position – the squat. Most people say they can't squat, but it's probably been a few years since they tried. You don't even have to try, but think about your seating. Its height is now your choice, as it is mine. We have control and can make changes. But first we have to be aware that there might be a problem.

I'll extend your choice and throw in a comfortable, squishy old sofa. You now have four seating arrangements to choose from. Which would you go for? I do hope you were very keen and said 'the squatting position on the telephone directories'. Good, I'll have that old sofa if you don't want it. There are no right or wrong answers!

—— Emotional contortionists ——

Time to watch television. I want you to curl up on that old squishy sofa, while you've still got it, and watch some soaps. Good old-fashioned soaps. You can choose which, but not your favourites that you watch all the time. Choose new soaps. Have a pen and paper handy and I want you to watch carefully. Not for a good plot or good or bad acting. I want you to watch for emotions and feelings. You know the sort of thing – anger, worry, love, joy, depression, confusion. All the range of emotions we humans have to go through. Watch what the actors do to express those feelings with their bodies. Especially, watch their heads and shoulders.

After you've watched for a while, I want you to turn off the television and try to imitate what you've seen.

Now I want you to act out those emotions yourself – you can do this privately in the bathroom if you prefer. Don't speak, just let your body act out how *you* feel when you're angry or happy or worried or thoughtful. See what your body does each time.

For the next few days I want you to watch yourself very carefully. As each of these feelings occurs naturally be aware and see how close to the actual body movement you were when you were alone in the bathroom. Did you get it right? Close? Or way out? How did the actors do?

Monitoring our feelings

Keep doing this. As the feelings occur monitor what you do with your body, and keep asking 'Why?' Now ask yourself what sparks off the feelings and whether they are valid. Did you get angry because the post was late? Were you anxious because someone promised to 'phone and they didn't? Did you feel elated because you thought you'd won the lottery and then felt depressed because you remembered you'd forgotten to buy a ticket?

All those feelings, all those body movements, what did any of it achieve? Did getting angry get the post to you any quicker? I think not. But it did increase your tension. What did you do with the tension afterwards?

Before we begin any body movement – and that includes being emotionally contorted – we can remember to *inhibit, project* and *control*. That way we don't need to respond to stimuli unnecessarily. That way we don't build up tension. That way we don't need to hold on to tension because we don't get it in the first place. That way we don't get out of alignment. Phew!

You made me do it

Let's clear up another popular misconception about feelings. Controlling our feelings does not make us robots: it makes us adults.

We can choose what we feel and the degree to which we feel it. 'Ah, I hear you say, 'but what if someone makes me angry?' That's the misconception. No-one can *make* you angry. They can do things that you can then choose to get angry about, but it's your choice: to have the feeling and then the degree to which you have it. But you'll say, 'what if something dreadful happens to someone I love – I'll feel sad.' Yes you will, but it's because you choose to, and sadness would be the right expression of your grief, just as anger might be the right expression for some other emotion. This isn't about not having feelings – it's about realising that we generate those feelings, that they are not visited upon us from some outside source. It's the stimulus that's outside and the feeling that's inside. The stimulus sparks off the feeling but we can choose not to respond to that stimulus, or to respond to a lesser degree, or be aware we have responded and then let go of the tension once we have done with it. If you got angry because the post was late and then went and killed the person who delivered it, that would be extreme, wouldn't it?

So where do you draw the line? How much anger is appropriate? Ask yourself that when you next get angry, and ask yourself what it achieves. This is about letting go of tension and not wasting energy.

What emotions are appropriate?

Suppose you come home and find someone has stolen everything you own. You'd certainly feel yourself do a perfect example of the startle pattern. And afterwards? What emotion or feeling would be appropriate? And to what degree? There are no *right* answers.

EXERCISE

Off to the bathroom with you again. I want you to stare at yourself in the mirror. Look closely at your eyes, don't let them move, and tell me the answer to the following questions:

1 What is 1394 divided by 7?
2 What is the capital of Thailand?
3 What's the biggest ocean in the world?

I don't want the answers. I want to know what your eyes did while you were working out the answers.

Now do it again and watch your eyes – don't let them move – and tell me the earliest memory you have. What did your eyes do?

Our eyes move when we think

If you refuse to allow your eyes to move, you may find it quite hard to work out the answers to anything. If your eyes did move they probably moved to the right and up while you worked out the answers to the first questions, and down and to the left while you told me about your childhood. This proves nothing except we move our eyes when we think. It's a neat party trick to play with friends.

The *primary control* is the head–neck relationship. The head is the primary control of the whole body, and the eyes are the primary control of the head. Our eyes are very important to our primary control, our primary control is very important to our movement, and our movement is important to our alignment. Where our eyes are directed can influence the position of our head which governs the rest of the body. Misdirect the eyes and the whole lot goes to pot. Direct the eyes and the whole lot comes together like a dream.

Go for a walk

Most people walk with their eyes looking down at their feet. This
leads the head to drop forwards, and the neck and back follow until
we have the often seen position – modern human (see Figure 6.2).

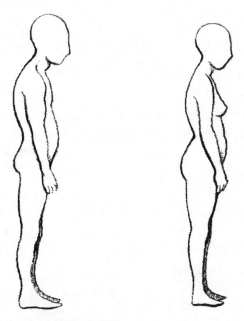

Figure 6.2   Modern man/woman

That's how most of us end up: bent, stooped, doubled up, call it what you want, it's a human form that's not aligned properly.

There are two ways we can avoid this. If I simply said, 'Stop watching your feet,' that would do little good. You might try for a while, but you actually need to learn a new way of walking.

A new way of walking

> ### EXERCISE
>
> I want you to take another walk and this time I want you to imagine that you are a robot from an alien planet. Inside your head there is not a brain or a mind but the most sophisticated and advanced computer in the universe. The computer has sensors that detect visual stimuli on the front surface of its mechanism. This robot is capable of 'seeing' and storing the visual images for long enough that it can 'remember' and not look again. As you walk, you can scan the ground ahead – about 3 m (10 feet) ahead of you. The computer will store all the information you need about surface texture, lumps and bumps, and unevenness. The computer will direct your feet and place them for you perfectly. I know this sounds silly but try it – all you have to do is trust.

You don't have to imagine that your head contains the most powerful computer in the universe; it does, your brain. Trust it. You don't have to bend over and peer at the ground when you walk. Try looking ahead and not at your feet. You'll find you can walk perfectly well, even better than before. We lose the art of trusting our natural instincts and instead try to control everything by conscious thought. Relax and let it work the way it was intended.

Walking with awareness

You can also try *walking with awareness*. Remember the exercise you did in Chapter 2 of noticing things that you had never seen before as you went into your home? Well you can expand that exercise and as you to walk everywhere begin to be aware of what is going on around you, above and ahead of you. Stroll and look without thought of what you have to do later, or what you're going to have for supper. Your walking will take no longer. In fact, you may even walk faster because you'll be walking more efficiently. Take time to notice what's happening all around you.

Why we walk the way we do

I bet if you got a piece of paper and a pen you could write down the names of all the members of your family and close friends and be able to describe in quite accurate detail things about the way they walk, what sort of stride they take, or the noise they make putting their feet down, or the speed of their walk. We recognise people at a distance by their walk long before we can make out their features. And we're just like them. We walk the same way all the time. We might speed up or slow down, but basically we walk in much the same way all the time. Now watch how a small child walks – he or she will walk a few steps, skip a few, jump a couple of times, run a bit, walk some more, hop on one leg for a while, turn around and walk backwards, hop again, skip and generally drive you mad. 'Walk properly!' 'Keep still!' 'Stop jigging about!' All instructions we've heard from our parents from time to time when we were small. We learn to control our natural urge to be constantly moving, constantly changing, and we learn to adopt a rigid and learnt habit or pattern of movement. We can try walking in different ways. How many different types of walk are there? You could take long strides, or short. A long stride with one leg and a short stride with the other. You could turn your feet in, or out, or one in and one out. You could take one fast step and one slow step. There are as many different ways of walking as there are people who walk. Why have we adopted only one? Try changing your walk. Try skipping or jumping.

True story

I was once giving a talk on the Alexander Technique to a large group of prison warders. One of them asked if I expected them to skip? 'Why not?' I replied, but I didn't think it was well received. A couple of weeks later I was back at the prison making arrangements for a follow-up lecture, and I asked the Assistant Governor how the first talk had gone. She said it was fine and that the next day a couple of prison warders had been seen skipping across the exercise yard. They had been applauded vigorously, by prisoners watching from the windows, whereupon they promptly held hands and skipped away. Apparently one of the prisoners later said that he thought it was brilliant – he hadn't realised the warders could be so human.

Puppets

As we walk we can imagine the string attached to the top of our heads pulling us up, holding and supporting us. This is not a movement: it is an imagining, a reprograming. Just the subtlest thought that will be buried deeply in your subconscious and which actually works – you'll walk more lightly.

EXERCISE

Go back to standing with your back to the wall. Let the three points of reference touch and keep your knees fairly straight. Now I want you to take just one step forwards and I want you to do it in slow motion. What happens? Did you lean slightly to one side as you lifted your leg to take that step? I bet you did. That's how most of us walk. We pick up each leg and throw it forwards and swivel our weight on to the forward leg while we pick up the back leg and throw that one forwards. A different way to try walking forwards, and one that is impossible to do in slow motion, is to take that first step by just letting yourself fall forwards. The weight of your head will act as a sort of pivot. You should find that this action makes you go up on to your toes and then you'll be obliged to take that first step without leaning to one side (see Figure 6.3). You'll be walking forwards as naturally as a small child does, falling into each new step.

Bouncing on your toes

Try walking around for a bit on tip-toe. Try bouncing on your toes as you walk. Try running by falling into the next step. Try standing in the narrowest doorway you can and take that first step. If you're doing it the new way you'll be fine, but if you're still doing it the old way you'll either touch the sides of the doorway, or you'll get stuck. If

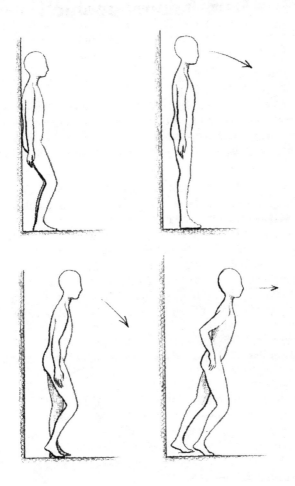

Figure 6.3   Taking the first step

you can't find a narrow enough doorway, try putting two poles in the ground in the garden, about the same width as your shoulders plus a little bit on each side. You could even try this just standing up against a wall. You'll lean to the side you start off on, so have the wall on that side.

───── Semi-supine position ─────

EXERCISE

For this exercise you will need a pen and paper and a friend. I want you to ask your friend if they will watch you carefully as you perform a simple action and record exactly how you do it: exactly where you put each limb, each bit of your body as you do it. Afterwards, you can keep this as a record of how you once did something and then we'll look at another way of doing it. Now go and get your friend.

I want you to place some books on the floor and stand next to them ready to get down into the *semi-supine position*. You only need a couple of books. I'll explain later how you can work out exactly how many and to what height. At the moment just have a few to prop up your head. From the standing position I want you to get down into the semi-supine while your friend records how you do it. You might, for instance, sit down first and then fall backwards, or squat down and then roll over into the position. Then I want you to get up again while your friend records that also. Again, for example, you might sit up, then stand up, or even, as I once saw, be able to spring completely upright by arching your back. Now you can thank your friend nicely and dispense with their services.

OK, so you've got your record – and I've seen some bizarre ways of getting down and up, so whatever you've got don't worry about it, it's just the way you used to do it. Now, I'm going to suggest a new way for you to do it. It's neither better nor worse, it's just new, and it puts a lot less strain on your body.

I'll go through it in stages. Then you can look at Figure 6.4 carefully, then *you* can try.

Getting down into the semi-supine position the new way

- **Stage 1** – Put the books on the floor and stand facing them a body's length away and one pace to the side of them. Let your arms hang loosely by your side and look straight ahead;

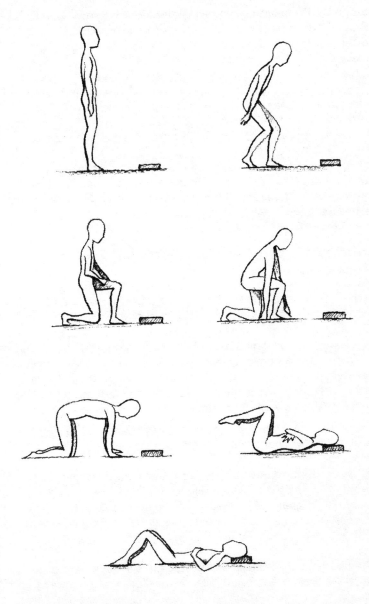

Figure 6.4 Getting down into the semi-supine position

- **Stage 2** – Bring one leg backwards until it is one stride behind;
- **Stage 3** – From this position drop down on to one knee;
- **Stage 4** – Lean forwards while still looking straight ahead and, using the arm that is opposite the knee that is still up, put that hand flat on the floor in front of you and to one side;
- **Stage 5** – Bring the other arm forwards and, as you do so, put the other knee flat on the floor until you are in the crawl position;
- **Stage 6** – Swing your bottom over towards the space in front of the book and let your body follow until you curl round into the semi-supine position with your knees bent;
- **Stage 7** – Check the books are in the right place, then adjust your arms so that they are in the right place with each hand either side on your lower stomach and the elbows on the floor. Make the 'ahhh' sound and relax.

Getting up from the semi-supine position in the new way

Basically it's the same, but in reverse, as getting down into the semi-supine with one additional point that is very important. We talked earlier about our eyes leading the movement. Well, in getting up from the semi-supine it is important to let our eyes lead us. First, though, we have to make a simple choice – which side to get up. We can get up to the right or to the left. It doesn't matter which, although it's important not to get into using one side as a habit – keep changing. Once we've made the decision we can get up (see Figure 6.5).

- **Stage 1** – Turn your eyes to the side you've chosen and let your head follow. As your head turns let your body follow and roll on to your side;
- **Stage 2** – Keep rolling until you are back in the crawl position;
- **Stage 3** – From the crawl position let your eyes lead the movement. You're going up, so that's where your eyes should be. Sink back on to your heels and, as you do so, bring your arms to your side with your finger tips just touching the floor and go up on to one knee;
- **Stage 4** – From one knee, still looking up and forwards, you can bring the other knee up and fall into your first step and away you go. Put your finger tips at the back of your neck for the first few times to make sure you aren't tempted to use your arms to lever yourself up from your knees.

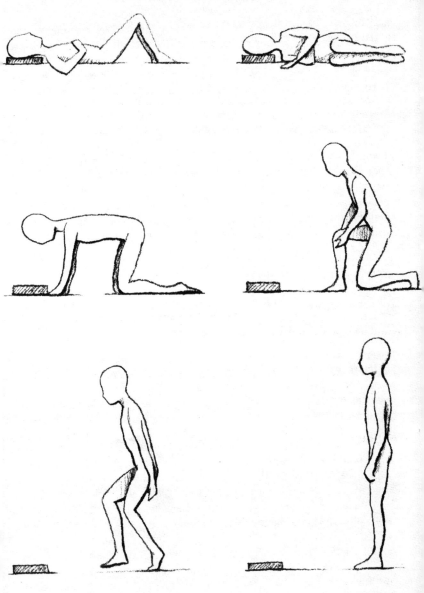

Figure 6.5   Getting up from the semi-supine position

Practise these new ways in slow motion until they become second nature. Eventually, your movements will become fluid and graceful. It doesn't put any strain or tension on any part of your body. Try this over the next few days and see how you get on. Remember, it's not better or worse, it's just new and less damaging.

When should we use the semi-supine?

Twice a day for fifteen minutes is really beneficial, but if you can't do that then I would recommend that you do it for fifteen minutes in the middle of the afternoon. We contract our muscles during the day as gravity takes its toll. By the middle of the afternoon we could do with *lengthening* again. Essentially, we shrink as the day goes on, and letting ourselves become taller again will restore our energy levels.

How many books?

You'll need your friend again. When you're lying in the semi-supine get him or her to check the height of your head. It should be parallel and level with your back, not at an angle up or down (see Figure 6.6).

What are we doing in the semi-supine?

You now know how to get down and up and how many books you need – but do you know what you're supposed to be doing while you're there? OK, your feet need to be positioned so that they are flat on the floor, parallel and about 50 cm (18 inches) apart. Your knees are bent and should be relaxed. If they have a tendency to fall outwards, move your feet slightly further apart. If they have a tendency to fall inwards, move your feet slightly closer together. Your hands should be relaxed and placed lightly one either side of your lower stomach. Your elbows should be touching the floor (see Figure 6.7). *Imagine* your whole torso lengthening and widening. Imagine yourself as liquid, about to flow into a relaxed puddle. The semi-supine position lets gravity work for a while in your favour. For so long it has been pulling you downwards, now you can use it to repair some of the damage it has caused. Gravity will pull your shoulders down into a more aligned position and help your back spread openly and widely.

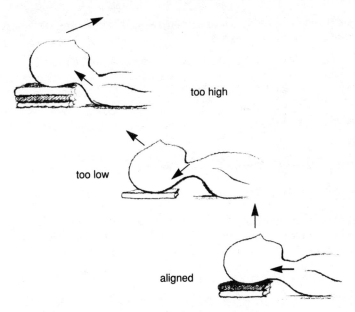

too high

too low

aligned

Figure 6.6   How to adjust the books for the semi-supine

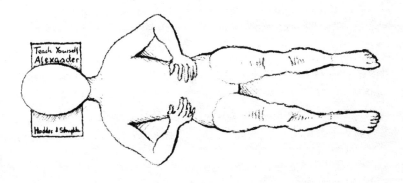

Figure 6.7   Semi-supine seen from above

Now sit up and lie down again to allow your back to lengthen. You may need to reposition the books.

If you want to know what your pelvis is doing while you are in this position, try putting your legs down flat on the floor and then bring them up again. Feel how your pelvis swivels and tilts backwards. That's a better alignment for it and one it gets little chance to use with modern living.

Using the semi-supine for relaxation

You may find holding this position quite exhausting at first: just lying there doing nothing can be tiring merely because it is strange. Some people find it very relaxing straight away and take to it immediately. I was one of those who found it tiring, and it took me several months to work up to fifteen-minute stretches. Now I find it tremendously relaxing. If I've been sitting working for a while and I'm getting tight around the shoulders, I will just stop for a bit, take up the semi-supine for a couple of minutes and feel all the tension leak away.

Summary

So now you know how to get down, get up and lie there in between. Use this position twice a day for fifteen minutes each time, or as long as you feel you can to begin with, and build up. If your knees get tired, you can put them down, but only one at a time and only for a few moments.

The semi-supine will correct a lot of misalignment, teach you a useful relaxation position and help your back to lengthen and widen.

In Chapter 7 we will look at how we can put the Alexander Technique into practical applications in our everyday life. But to summarise those topics we have looked at in this chapter:

- defining the Alexander Technique
- misconceptions about *inhibiting, conscious projecting* and *primary control*
- the best **use** of ourselves
- realigning ourselves
- how we get out of alignment

- choosing our seating position
- how our emotions can change our body shape
- a new way of walking
- the *semi-supine*.

Conclusions

- We need to be constantly adapting and changing;
- We need to be aware of how much we move by habit and, if those habits are not done according to the best principles of body design, change them.

7

PRACTICAL
APPLICATIONS

I may be mistaken in my belief that everything you do is wrong, in which case you would be doing the right thing to ignore me.

F M Alexander

Alexander developed his technique originally because he wanted to do something – put on his one-man show without losing his voice. The Technique, to him, was a tool. It enabled him to carry on with his career. It was only later that he became a teacher. He developed the Technique to be of use, and that's how it works best, when it just sits there in the background helping you to function more efficiently than before. Under ideal conditions, you shouldn't be aware that it's even there.

The operating system

In Chapter 3 we talked about the *three stages of doing*. In ideal circumstances, the Alexander Technique in operation should be Stage 4. In case you've forgotten the four stages, here they are again:

- **Stage 1** – Unconscious inefficiency
- **Stage 2** – Conscious inefficiency
- **Stage 3** – Conscious efficiency
- **Stage 4** – Unconscious efficiency

And we also talked about the three ways of doing something:

- the way you would do it without thinking
- the way you would do it if you were thinking
- the way it's designed to be done

So by now we ought to be at about Stage 2. We know we're not doing as we were designed to do. And maybe we are also beginning to do things more consciously. When I first learnt about the Alexander Technique I was told to monitor everything I did for the next week or so and write down *how* I did every action. I want you to do the same with the following provisos: that you also explain *why* you do anything; and that you fill in a chart. This may make it a lot easier for you to record the positions of the parts of the body, as well as help you to remember to do this, and it is also useful as a record you can look back on later.

EXERCISE

Use the chart to record certain actions, as you do them; if this is not possible, write them up afterwards from memory. There are some blank action spaces for you to fill in, in case you have a special occupation, hobby, activity or whatever that is not listed. Remember, there are no right answers – it's not a test. All you have to do is answer as accurately as you can, and as honestly as you can. This is an exercise to get you thinking not only about how you move your body, but also, more importantly, *why* you move it in the way you do.

Filling in your chart

How much detail you want to go into depends on how effective you want to be. By not being aware of what we are doing with our bodies we cannot hope to make improvements. By watching and correcting we can learn a new way of *doing* that will require far less effort, be more relaxing, allow us to move with more grace, free us from aches and pains, eliminate potentially harmful habits and improve our physical, emotional and mental well being. Not a bad result for just a little observation and practice. Believe me, it all becomes much easier once the basic principles are second nature. The Alexander Technique requires a new way of looking at body movement. Each *doing* should be accompanied by: 'What am I doing? Am I doing in the way the body

	Body part							
Activity	Left hand	Right hand	Left arm	Right arm	Head	Neck	Shoul-ders	Back
Washing up								
Getting into bed								
Getting out of bed								
Cleaning teeth								
Watching TV								
Driving car								
At work								
Walking								
Sitting down								
Sitting								
Standing up								
Lifting objects								

	Torso	Hips	Right thigh	Left thigh	Right calf	Left calf	Right foot	Left foot	**Reason for body shape**

is designed to do? How can I improve my doing?' When you get into the way of checking how you move it becomes part of your life quickly. Filling in the chart is a way of getting you to look at how you carry out everyday routines. Once you've looked at it you may realise at once that you are using too much effort, or too much tension, or using the muscles or just moving with faulty motivation (end gaining).

Example 1 – Watching television

Let's take a common example like sitting watching television. I'll assume it's something we all do from time to time. Don't try to do anything different, just do it the way you normally would and monitor how you do it. Remember, there is no right or wrong so be as honest as you can. On page 108 you will see how I have filled in my chart.

I have used my own codes, but the chart gives me a good idea of how I slump to watch television. Now I've had a look at this, I can determine what's wrong. If my TV set is on the floor then I have to lean my head forwards to see it. My eyes lead the movement. Once my head is

Here is the chart that I filled in when I was watching television:

	Body part							
Activity	Left hand	Right hand	Left arm	Right arm	Head	Neck	Shoul-ders	Back
Watching TV	under chin	in lap	bent	loose	down left	over to left	left up	lean to left

Here is the chart that I filled in when I was sweeping:

	Body part							
Activity	Left hand	Right hand	Left arm	Right arm	Head	Neck	Shoul-ders	Back
Sweeping	low grip	high grip	low tense	high tense	down front	over to front	tense	bent tense

down then my neck and back have to follow – primary control. I'm not aligned as well as I could be, so the whole lot goes to pot. I start using my arms to prop up my head instead of it resting naturally, supported by my neck which should be supported by my back. When I start using my arms – activity muscles – I get tired quickly, which means I slump even more. Solution? Easy – put the TV set at a height where my eyes look straight ahead, then my head will be aligned, my back straight, my arms not needed for supporting anything (see Figure 7.1). Result? I can relax and feel more rested, which is why I was trying to relax and watch television in the first place.

Example 2 – Sweeping

I find that when I'm sweeping I have a tendency to hunch over, grip the broom handle far tighter than is really necessary, use a lot of muscular power from my arms and bend my head down too far. If I straighten up I start to use the muscular power of my back which is far less exhausting and the whole posture is aligned (see Figure 7.2).

Torso	Hips	Right thigh	Left thigh	Right calf	Left calf	Right foot	Left foot	**Reason for body shape**
sag to left	left tight	↙	↘	↓	↓	over left	on floor	TV on floor so need to look downwards

Torso	Hips	Right thigh	Left thigh	Right calf	Left calf	Right foot	Left foot	**Reason for body shape**
bent tense	straight	↓	↓	↓	↓	for-wards	on floor	Need to look down to see what I am sweeping

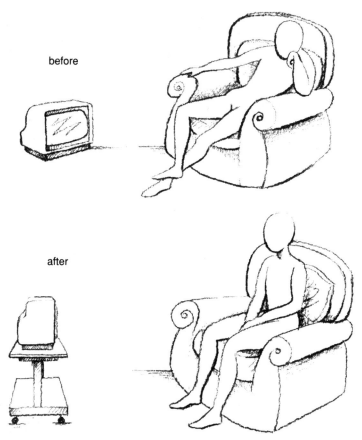

Figure 7.1 Watching television

Emotional tensions

Spend some time over the next week or so just running through your daily activities to see how you do them. If they are activities you do regularly, there will undoubtedly be habits that go with them. You can also check the emotional posture you adopt – does having to do the washing-up set up emotional tension? You may not even be aware of it until you observe yourself closely. You may feel resentful – it's not your turn or you might feel you're being taken for granted –

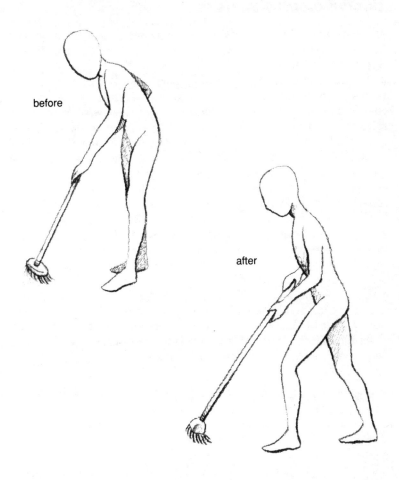

before

after

Figure 7.2 Sweeping - mis-aligned and aligned

and you'll tense up. Or there may be some past emotional resentment still lurking – every time you have to put the rubbish out, you find yourself strangely tense: you do it in a well-aligned way, but there is still tension. Then you remember how your father always made you put the rubbish out before you could have your pocket money and you're still hanging on to that resentment. It does happen.

Unconscious signals

As we perform our tasks we are also giving off signals about how we feel by the body posture we adopt. In most cases these signals will be fine, but occasionally they will convey information that we might not intend, or they might be conveying information that is accurate but that we don't want revealed. It is also useful when you fill in your chart to imagine how you must appear to other people, or watch yourself in a mirror while you are *doing*. I'll give you an example of what is meant by *unconscious signals*. I was at an Alexander Technique workshop once where we were mimicking each other's walk. It was all quite fun, but there was a young man there who had been through a lot in his life – in trouble with the police, bullied, mugged, robbed and generally one of life's victims. His walk seemed to reflect his troubles. He held himself in a permanent hunched position as if expecting the next blow. At the end of the workshop we were told to go home practising some one else's walk as an experiment. One chap elected to copy the young man's walk and on the way home was stopped by the police, set upon and chased by a crowd of hooligans and he also managed to lose his wallet. Coincidence? Maybe, but what comes first? Did the young man's walk come from his troubles? Or were his troubles attracted to him by his demeanour. Oh yes, the other chap was a policeman himself, and even he said it was quite scary how frightened and unsure of himself he felt when he was mimicking the young man's walk.

The young man had mimicked the policeman's walk that night and had experienced no trouble at all – and he did say he felt more confident, more powerful and more in control of himself than ever before. It took quite a lot of persuading to stop him trying to adopt the policeman's walk permanently. He was eventually convinced of the importance of finding his own walk, and he managed to adopt a more aligned and more upright walk.

Thinking ahead

Working through our chart we will become aware of how often the correction to our misalignment seems to be a subtle adjustment to our head's position. We can help our head find an alignment that is better for it if we *think a head, ahead*. If we are giving our head a hard time it won't align well. Take how we sleep for example. How many pillows do you use? And why? Your pillow height should be the same as the book height when you're in the semi-supine position if you lie on your back. But if lying on your side, you will need more pillow. Take a look at Figure 7.3 to see why.

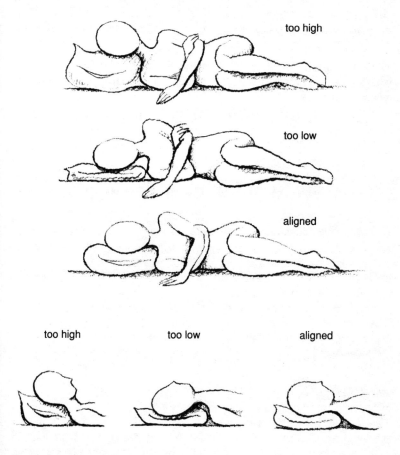

too high

too low

aligned

too high   too low   aligned

Figure 7.3   Pillow height

Get it straight

Once we've checked the height of our heads, we can check the height of our eyes. The straighter our eyes, the straighter our heads. I used to watch television with the TV set on the floor. I now have it at head height and find it a much more aligned, relaxed and comfortable position.

It's surprising how many people use computers and have the screen offset to one side and at a height lower than their eye-line. If you have to sit there and stare at a screen all day, then it should be in front of you and at the same height as your eyes.

The same applies if you go to the cinema – it's better to choose a seat where you don't have to turn your head to look up, or crane to look down.

I'm sure that as you get used to checking your alignment you'll find lots of examples of your own where you've adopted a poor alignment due to not keeping straight.

—— How to enjoy exercise more ——

I used to hate to exercise. I got hot. I got tired. I got miserable. But it was surprising how many times I used the wrong muscles to exercise the wrong bits. I'm not suggesting that you *have* to exercise – you don't *have* to do anything – but if you apply the principles you've learnt, you may find that any exercise – jogging, swimming, bicycling – gets easier and more enjoyable. If you practise yoga or Tai Ch'i you may find that your movements become more fluid and effortless if you take some time to incorporate the principles of the Alexander Technique.

Motivation in middle age

There's a natural tendency to sag as we get older – gravity is pretty powerful stuff. As we sag, we lose our body shape which makes us look baggy and older. The older and more lifeless we look, the older and more lifeless we're going to feel. The older we feel, the less likelihood there is of us doing anything about it. Down we go. Finding the incentive to do something about the decline can be quite hard. The Alexander Technique restores our poise without us having to do very much at all. Once our poise returns we start to look better.

Looking better and feeling better become the same thing. Once we feel better, we are more inclined to have the energy and motivation to do something about the decline. Up we go. A lot of people who have practised the Alexander Technique have lived to incredible old age and, while I wouldn't like to promote the Alexander Technique as a passport to longevity, I am convinced of its power to motivate us into feeling and being fitter and more active. If we don't lose the energy in the first place, we'll have a *head* start from the beginning.

A pain in the neck

When I first started the Alexander Technique I had a friend, or rather an acquaintance, who would drop round and borrow things and never return them, outstay his welcome, irritate me in a thousand different ways and generally be a *pain in the neck*. It had never dawned on me that that's exactly what he was, a pain in the neck – my neck. Practising the Alexander Technique gave me the confidence – and desire for self-preservation – to tell this sponger to 'get lost'. I'd realised that whenever a visit was threatened, I found myself getting extremely tense, especially round the shoulders and neck – a literal pain in the neck. I'd always put up with it, now I realised the physical damage it was causing I was able to be assertive enough to cancel the intrusion and feel a whole lot better afterwards.

—— Thinking for ourselves ——

It would be terribly easy to take you through all the everyday activities that we subject our bodies to and *tell* you the *right* way and the *wrong* way in which they should all be done. However, that would achieve nothing. You'd then have a fixed idea of *right* and *wrong* which wouldn't help at all. The only *right* is doing something in the manner for which the body was designed – the *means whereby*. All the rest is choice.

I recently read a book on the Alexander Technique that said you mustn't cross your legs when you're sitting down. That, I think is your choice. You can cross them or not. The only *right* thing is to be aware of what is wrong when we perform in a way which will cause damage or be inefficient. You have to do some work yourself, you know.

Summary

So to summarise this chapter:

- fill in your chart – be honest and as accurate as you can
- analyse each activity for poor alignment – What could you change? What could you improve? What do you do through habit?
- unconscious signals – see if you're giving off any; they may affect the way people react to you
- think a *head* – your head is important so give it some attention
- try to keep your eyes straight – by starting off straight, we end up straight.

In Chapter 8 we'll look at the anatomy of the human body and how it works well when it's aligned according to its design principles.

8
THE BODY EXPLAINED

The old idea of trying to be right has stayed with us in spite of the fact that conditions have changed – and our right is wrong.

F M Alexander

If we have a faulty idea of how the body works, we cannot hope to be able to put 'right' what is 'wrong'. A lot of people have a confused notion of how we manage to stand up in the first place and how, and even where, the head is balanced on the spinal column.

The spinal column

In nearly all people, although there are exceptions, the spinal column is made up of thirty-three *vertebrae* (the bones that make up the spine) joined together by *discs* (joints which allow us to carry out various forms and amounts of movement). While there is movement between the individual joints, the whole structure is usually seen as a whole – rather like a pile of children's wooden bricks balanced on top of each other with a thin layer of rubber sandwiched in between each one. If you put weight on the top of it the rubber compresses and the whole structure gets shorter. Take the weight off and the whole thing elongates again.

The head

The head is balanced on top of the spinal column and is offset towards the front. It is balanced at a point just behind the ears. A lot of people, if you ask them where they think the head is balanced, will usually point to their neck, but the pivot point is much higher. The head balances freely on top of the spine on the *atlanto-occipital* joint – this means it sits on the *atlas vertebra* supported by the the occipital bone at the bottom of the skull. The bulk of the skull is carried forwards of the atlanto-occipital joint so various muscles are needed to support its weight (see Figure 8.1).

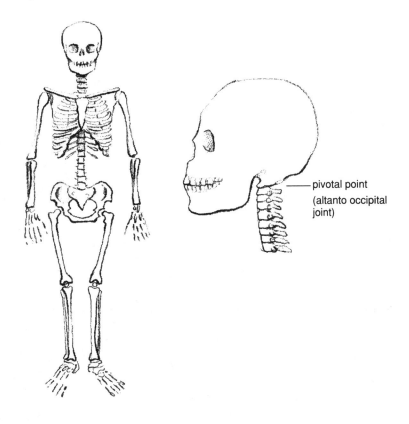

pivotal point
(altanto occipital
joint)

Figure 8.1   Head, neck - skeletal

The back

The ribs are attached to the upper part of the back at the *thoracic vertebrae*. The ribs enclose the lungs, heart, stomach and other important organs such as the liver, and are held together by muscle which also connect them to the spine, pelvis, shoulders and arms. These muscles, working in conjunction with the *diaphragm* (which is the muscular bit that separates the chest from the abdomen), allow the ribs movement. It is these muscles which are frequently held in tension – this causes us to have restricted rib movement which reduces our capacity for breathing and interferes with all the major organs. By allowing the back, especially the ribs, to *widen* we can recover the lost movement with all its inherent benefits. There are nine groups of muscles in the neck alone and thirty-two groups in the back. When we contract these muscles by misalignment or by *doing* wrongly, we contort the whole structure in a way it wasn't designed to be held. However, we cannot recover their elongation by *doing*; only by *not doing* can we relax them and thus gain benefit.

Muscles

All your muscles are made up of fibres and nerves. The individual nerve cells are called *motor-neurones* and every single one of them starts in the spinal column. The nerve connections, *axones*, extend from the spinal column to the muscle fibres. The muscle is contracted by an electrical impulse that is sent from the brain, down the spinal column, along the axones and to the muscle motor mechanisms. Essentially, the muscles are contracted by signals sent from our brain, which is where we think.

Research has shown that we can improve our performance in anything from playing darts to basketball shooting merely by imagining that our performance has improved. By going through the mental process, without practising it physically, we already train the muscles to respond naturally when we call upon them to act out in real life that for which we have trained them in our imagination. They have already received the signals.

Lengthening

The muscles that hold the spine in shape can be contracted and held under tension in much the same way as the muscles which hold the ribs in shape – and the same rule applies. You can contract them by *doing*, but only by *not doing* can you release them. There is no movement that can release muscles. Release comes from letting go of any trigger mechanisms that fire in the muscles causing them to contract. We cannot unfire by doing. We can only not do and thus cause release and relaxation. Not doing is harder than doing because we have lost the art of not doing. If you want to test just how hard it is, try this simple test of not doing. Hold up one of your hands at waist height with the other hand. The hand holding up lets go of the other hand and it has to drop just as if it were a dead thing. How did yours drop – if it did at all? Mostly we find that *letting go* is one of the hardest things to do, because we think of it as something to do rather than not do.

Moving without moving

Try another test. As you are reading this, become aware of the index finger of your left hand. Ask yourself in what direction it is pointing and see what it is pointing at. Look at what it is pointing at without moving your head or your finger. Concentrate really hard on whatever your finger is pointing at and imagine your finger pointing at it even more. I bet that you cannot help but move your finger, no matter how hard you try not to. Merely by concentrating – and issuing no instructions to move – we move.

Muscle has a very rich blood supply and, because of this, can remain relatively free from infection. The fibres of the involuntary muscles are finer and smaller than those of the voluntary muscles. It takes about a hundredth of a second to fire the trigger that causes a muscle to contract and it can, when and if required, support a thousand times its own weight. Powerful stuff. If you over use a muscle, it loses its ability to contract for a while. If permanently over-used, it can lose the ability indefinitely.

Nerves

Nerves are to be found in every part of our bodies. There is no part that is not in some way sensitive to pain or other sensations. The nervous system is usually considered to have two parts: the *peripheral* or outside – the part of the nerve that comes into contact with the stimuli that causes it to react, such as temperature or pain – and the *central system* which is made up of the spinal cord and the brain. The spinal cord is the part that runs up inside the spinal column and carries all the messages to the brain. It's obviously an important pathway, and you can see that any excess compression or distortion of the spine is likely to interfere with this pathway.

Bones

Essentially, all the bones that make up our limbs are either hanging from or attached in some way to the spine. The bones are held together at the joints by *ligaments* which are made of tough rope-like strands of tissue. Inside each joint is a thin bag of membrane which secretes a lubricant to make the joint move smoothly. Some joints slide over each other, such as the lower jaw moving over the upper; others are hinged like the elbows and knees; others are made of a ball and socket arrangement like the hips. Some bones are permanently fused together like the five large lower vertebrae, the *sacrum*.

There are various types of bones: long ones for levering and flat ones that are essential for muscle action. They don't stop growing until we are between fifteen and twenty-five years old. You can see how essential positive alignment is in children if they are to grow to their full potential.

The holistic approach

The human body is a complex and fascinating mechanism that lasts with minimum maintenance for our entire life. Yet, how many of us give it a single thought during our normal everyday life? It is a system that is so interconnected that the merest change to one thing within that system causes reactions with the entire system. We cannot isolate any part and expect it to function independently. If the system is misaligned it will be unable to function efficiently. If that inefficiency is allowed to become habit it will affect not only our posture, with its manifestations as aches and pains, but also our respiratory, digestive, emotional and mental facilities. Correct the physical misalignment and the entire system improves and begins to function smoothly and naturally, with an ease and grace of performance in all areas of our lives.

—— How the Technique can help us ——

In Chapter 7 we looked at some daily activities that the Alexander Technique can help with. I would now like to look at a few more. Some of these are the activities that teachers of the Alexander Technique get asked about more often than anything else. We'll look at how these activities, when done in a misaligned way, can throw the whole system out and cause us to function inefficiently in areas other than the purely physical, such as digestive or respiratory.

Children

Being around children can teach us a lot, but it can also be a source of misalignment. Children have to be carried, changed and generally looked after. They are heavy and we can develop some unfortunate habits if we don't think about what we are doing. Lifting children, especially out of cots, can be damaging. Changing babies' nappies can also be detrimental if we adopt habits without thinking about them. In both cases, it's important to remember that your back works best when kept straight. If you think of your back as the *motor* and your arms as the *controls*, you can see that if you keep your back straight you have full use of the motor, and can then use the controls to direct the activities with less energy being expended (see Figure 8.2).

Car driving

We are funny things, we humans. We have a perfectly good means of getting around, but we have to try to go faster. Driving cars, while it

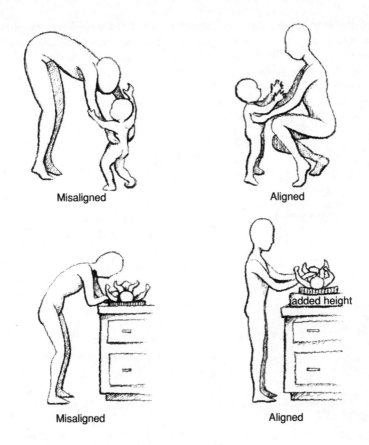

Misaligned

Aligned

Misaligned

Aligned

added height

Figure 8.2 Lifting babies and changing nappies

may be convenient and quick, can be a source of misalignment. The average seats in a car are exactly that – average. We, however, are not. We come in all shapes and sizes and the seats weren't designed for us individually. Remember, we talked about keeping our feet flat on the floor? In a car that's impossible if you are the driver because you have to raise one foot permanently to operate the accelerator and brake, while the other foot is raised and lowered intermittently to operate the clutch pedal. That's why long car journeys can be so exhausting – we use our activity muscles in our arms to hold us up after a while. Look carefully at the way you drive and see if you don't sag quickly and end up using the steering wheel to pull yourself forwards. Most people also have the seat raked at an angle. It might be an improvement if we were to sit up straighter and put a wedge cushion under our bottoms (see figure 8.3). For information about cushions see 'Useful Information'.

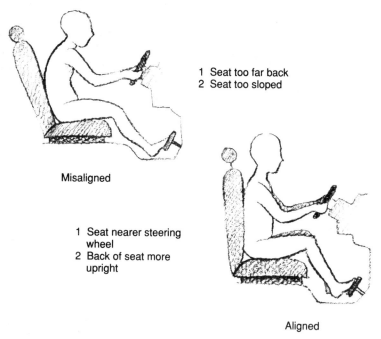

1 Seat too far back
2 Seat too sloped

Misaligned

1 Seat nearer steering wheel
2 Back of seat more upright

Aligned

Figure 8.3   Sitting in a car

Sitting at a desk

I know we've covered this before, but it's an important aspect of our daily lives. We might not be sitting at a desk to work, but we do sit at tables to eat and the same principles of improved alignment apply equally well.

Sitting, as we found out, is not really a natural human activity – squatting is where it's at. If you can't squat, you practise. If you have to hold on to something to be able to get down into the squatting position, then hold on until it becomes easier and you get used to it. It's not natural to lose the ability to squat as we get older: I know you'll probably think it is, but it isn't. The habit of losing abilities is just that – a habit. There is no reason why we can't continue all physical activities all of our lives. If we have to sit for long periods, we need to think about our sitting position. Try to keep your feet flat on the floor, use a wedge cushion if you don't want to take a saw to the front legs of the chair (see Figure 8.4). Keep everything you need for your work on the opposite side of the room from your desk. 'But that's crazy,' I hear you say, 'I need it all at my desk, don't I?' Well, yes you need it, but you also need to move around as much as you sit. By having to get up to fetch your stapler or paperclips you'll stop yourself getting stiff from sitting for too long.

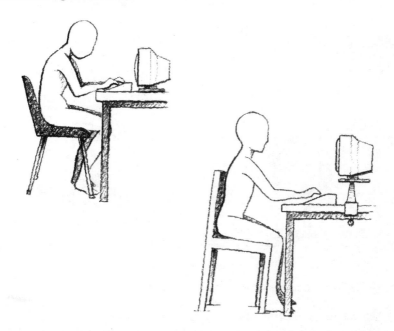

Figure 8.4 Sitting at a desk

Make sure your desk is high enough to be able to reach everything without having to bend over.

You can even try the *Balans* chair (see Figure 8.5). This is designed so that you can sit with your feet flat on the floor and your knees supported as well as keeping your back straight. It also helps to transfer

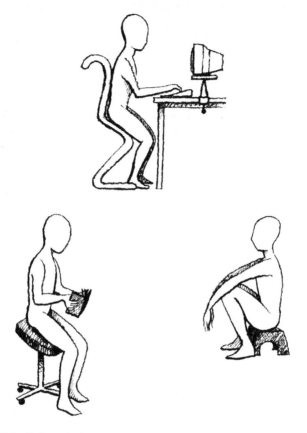

Figure 8.5   Balans chair and improved sitting positions

the weight away from your pelvis, which makes it easier to sit for long periods (see 'Useful Information'). Also remember that your ideal sitting position is the squat. At times during the day it is beneficial to squat down, or at least get your knees up by placing your feet on a high pile of books or directories.

Standing, walking, running, jumping

A useful exercise is to look through books and magazines of different ethnic types of peoples. We come in all shapes and sizes, colours and types. What we have in common is that we are all human and, as such, have the same potential for alignment and misalignment. If you look at different ethnic groups you'll see how some people seem to have a natural poise and grace, while others seem somehow contorted and weighed down – especially Westerners. Most people who live a simpler, more natural existence seem to move with a gentle grace and balance that Westerners have lost. By studying pictures of other types of people we can identify what it is about them that gives them their fluid movements. Often we may spot the fact that they are barefoot The feet are designed to be placed flat on the ground and any change in this basic good design can't be helpful. We have natural soft soles on our feet to absorb impact and be resistant to shocks and strains. Any attempt to interfere with this softness causes us problems. We need our feet to retain their natural flexibility. We have around twenty-six bones in each foot and they shouldn't be restricted if we are to maintain a good balance. Constricting our feet also causes us to transfer any side-to-side balancing upwards to the knees. The knee joint is designed to flex front and back with some rotary movement – it has little side-to-side movement, so that movement may be transferred further up to your hips. The higher you go, the greater the side-to-side balancing movements become. This causes some people to sway noticeably as they walk.

Footwear

Obviously we can't go barefoot with as much social ease as some peoples but we can go barefoot as much as possible at home – and try to wear soft-soled, low-heeled shoes out of doors.

High heels have three major disadvantages: they put too much pressure on the arch of your foot, make you throw too much weight on to the front of your foot, and stop any effective gripping action of the toes. But don't stop wearing them just because I seem to have a negative response to them – you must decide for yourself. If you do decide to stop wearing them, it is advisable to lower your heels over a period of some weeks gradually, rather than going from high heels to flat shoes immediately. That would put too much strain on contorted ligaments in your legs and back. We have to undo the damage slowly.

Hard soles also have their problems: we can't grip with our toes as well, the foot cannot shape itself to uneven surfaces as well which makes it overbalance on rough ground, and we can't bend properly at the ankle.

Our feet are important. We need to be able to balance, grip with our toes, maintain flexibility and absorb impact. Do your shoes let you do all that?

Toilets

Tricky subject this, but we all have to use them. Why are they the height and shape they are? To fit your bottom? I think not. They are uniformly made for ease of manufacture - and three-quarters of the worlds population doesn't use them. They are used mostly in the West and it might be interesting some time to compare the statistics for bowel cancer with those of more simple living peoples. Bowel cancer is very prevalent in the West and I'm not suggesting for one moment that it's down to toilet design, but if we are not using our bowels properly they can only malfunction. We are designed to squat – that's all there is to it. Squatting allows us to pass larger stools, empty our bowels more completely and supports the stomach muscles. If you want to try, you can squat or raise your legs by resting them on a box or pile of books.

You can even try squatting on the toilet itself (see Figure 8.6). This may sound odd or unusual to Westerners, but not so to some people. A friend was working on a ship that had a large contingent of Chinese crew. He said that the Chinese used to laugh at the way the Westerners used the toilet, just as much as the Westerners laughed at the Chinese. The Westerners used it in a conventional fashion while the Chinese squatted on the seat. Which way is better? Which way is right?

Conscious choice

There are no right or wrong answers to any of this – there is only choice. Until you think consciously about how you do everything, you can't make choices. Once you can, you are freed from habits. It's the habits that causes the problems – not that they are necessarily wrong. It is essential to be flexible in our routines and flexible in our bodies. When we have a set way of doing something we no longer think about how we do it – thus we become rigid, physically and mentally.

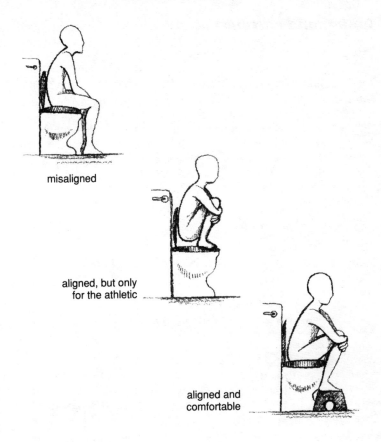

misaligned

aligned, but only
for the athletic

aligned and
comfortable

Figure 8.6 Toilet sitting

Sex and the Alexander Technique

Another tricky subject this. Having sex probably uses more of our
body than any other activity, but how often do we think about using
our bodies to their best during sex? You should have picked up
enough pointers from this book as you've got this far, so I will leave it
to you to practise. If you want to learn more, there is an excellent
book on the subject: *Sexuality and the Alexander Technique* by Chloe
Stallibrass (available from STAT Books).

Lifting and carrying

Our arms and hands are for pointing to what we want in shops, our backs are for carrying it home. We all mix these two up. Keeping your back straight controls the flexing of the lumbar region and stabilises the pelvic area. Did you know that your spine has over a hundred muscle attachments? Those muscle attachments all work to help you lift and carry. Ideally, we should aim to carry loads equally distributed on both sides of our body. How often have you seen someone struggling to carry one over-full carrier bag of shopping when two

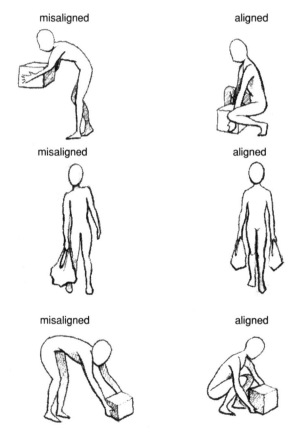

misaligned   aligned

misaligned   aligned

misaligned   aligned

Figure 8.7   Lifting and carrying

bags would have made more sense? Or people with a briefcase or suit-case that was too heavy, pulling them over to one side? Or people car-rying heavy parcels under their arms when they could have carried them on their shoulders?

If you have to lift heavy objects from the floor it is important to keep flexible. Lift with your back and keep your knees bent. Don't bend over from the waist with stiff knees – that's not the way it's designed to be done. Try squatting down to pick things up, or try putting one foot slightly in front of the other to give yourself more grip on the ground. (see Figure 8.7).

Lifting ourselves

Throughout the day we spend a lot of time lifting ourselves up. This starts first thing in the morning when we lift ourselves out of bed. If we use gravity, and the power and strength of a straight back, we can stop wasting energy lifting ourselves using our arms. Every time you have to lift yourself – from sitting or lying – try using the weight of your head to pivot yourself up. Or you can roll in and out of bed, or kneel to get up and down into a lying position.

Getting out of the bath

This is another example of how the principles of the Alexander Technique can be useful. We all know how difficult it can be to get out of the bath at times – we're wet and it's an awkward position to rise from. However, if you try this you may find it a lot easier. From the lying down position try rolling on to your side. Then continue the roll until you are in the crawl position. From the crawl position you can kneel, and then on to one knee. Once on one knee you can stand up with minimal effort (see Figure 8.8). Try it, but be careful not to slip or injure yourself. I think you'll find it a lot easier than the conventional hauling yourself up using your arms.

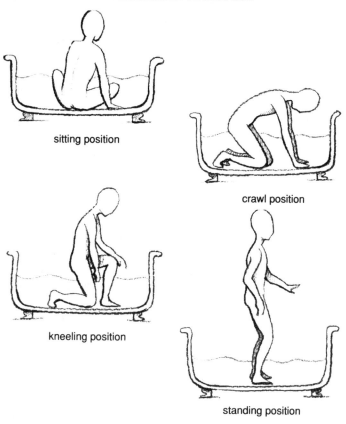

sitting position

crawl position

kneeling position

standing position

Figure 8.8 Getting out of the bath using the Alexander Technique

Summary

I'm not going to summarise this chapter – that would just be habit. I hope that this book has gone a long way to explaining the Alexander Technique and that you find learning it as helpful as many thousands of people before you. There are only three basic principles I would remind you about:

● let the neck be free
● let the head go forwards and up
● allow the back to lengthen and widen.

Apart from that, it's up to you. Good luck and stay flexible.

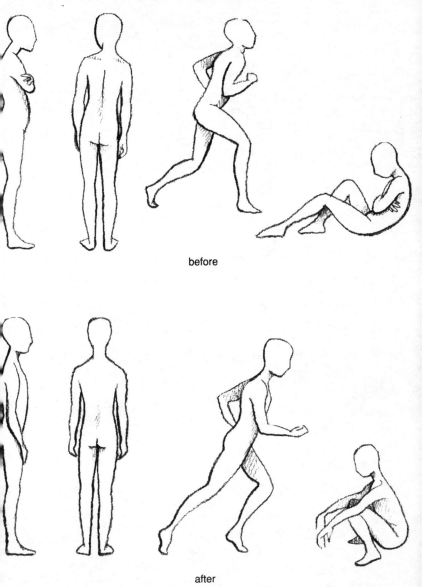

before

after

Figure 8.9 Before and after the Alexander Technique

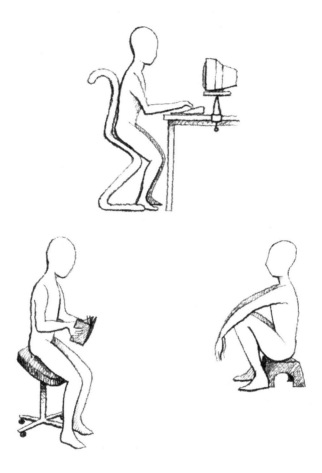

Figure 8.10   After the Alexander Technique

The difficulty for us all is to take up a new way of life in which we must apply principles instead of the haphazard end-gaining methods of the past. This indicates a slow process and we must all be content with steady improvements from day to day; but we must see to it that we are really depending upon the application of our principles in all our endeavours in every direction from day to day. You have been too anxious to be right despite the fact that you learnt early in your lessons that your right was wrong. However you have done well considering your difficulties, and you will continue to improve in the controlled use of yourself if you work as steadily as directed.

F M Alexander

USEFUL INFORMATION

Be careful of the printed matter; you may not read it as it was written.

F M Alexander

If you want to write to any of the addresses listed here for further details please enclose a stamped self-addressed envelope – many of these organisations are staffed by volunteers and are run on donations and contributions.

If you want to know more about the Society of Teachers of the Alexander Technique (STAT) you can become an *Associate Member*. It will keep you up to date with news of developments in the Technique, send you copies of the Society newsletter, STAT News, three times a year, and inform you of the Annual Conference, which you will be allowed to attend, where you can meet teachers and other students. You will also be sent a list of teachers, a catalogue of STAT Books and a free invitation to attend the F M Alexander memorial lecture which takes place annually. You will need to be proposed by a full member, such as a qualified teacher, and it will cost you £15 per year.

Addresses of the Society worldwide

United Kingdom

STAT, The Society of Teachers of the Alexander Technique
20 London House
266 Fulham Road
London SW10 9EL

Australia

Australian Society of Teachers of the Alexander Technique
(AUSTAT)
PO Box 716
Darlinghurst
NSW 2010

Canada
Canadian Society of Teachers of
the Alexander Technique
(CANSTAT)
PO Box 47025
19 – 555 West 12th Avenue
Vancouver

Denmark
Danish Society of Teachers of the
Alexander Technique (DFLAT)
c/o Marc Grue
Secretary
Otto Ruds Gade 38 st. th.
DK – 8200 Aarhus

International School for the
FM Alexander Technique
J. Berthelsenv. 15A
9400 Norresundby

Germany
German Society of Teachers of
the Alexander Technique (GLAT)
Postfach 5312
79020 Freiburg

Israel
Israeli Society of Teachers of the
Alexander Technique (ISTAT)
c/o Gideon Avrahami
Kibbutz Ein-Sheme M P
Menashe 37845

Netherlands
Alexander Technick Opeiding
Nedrland
Greef Aelbrechtlaan 6
1181 SW Amstelveen

Alexander Technique Centre
Amsterdam
340 Herengracht
1016 CG Amsterdam

South Africa
South African Society of
Teachers of the Alexander
Technique (SASTAT)
35 Thornhill Road
Rondebosch 7700

Switzerland
Swiss Society of Teachers of the
Alexander Technique (SVLAT)
Postfach CH 8032
Zurich

USA
North American Society of
Teachers of the Alexander
Technique (NASTAT)
PO Box 517
Urbana
IL 61801-0517

There are also teachers in Austria, Belgium, Brazil, Colombia, Eire, Finland, France, Hong Kong, Iceland, India, Italy, Japan, Luxembourg, Malaysia, Mexico, New Zealand, Norway, Poland, Singapore, Spain, Sweden, and the Seychelles. A list of qualified teachers in these countries can be obtained from STAT.

Other useful addresses

The Alexander Institute
16 Balderton Street
London W1Y YTF

Alexander Research Trust
18 Lansdowne Road
London W11 3LL

The Alexander Teaching Centre
188 Old Street
London EC1V 9BP

Alexander Technique Training
Centre
Community College
Fore Street
Totnes
Devon TQ9 5RP

The Centre for the Alexander
Technique
46 Stevenage Road
London SW6 6HA

The Centre for Development in
Alexander Technique
142 Thorpedale Road
London N4 3BS

The Constructive Teaching
Centre
18 Lansdowne Road
London W11 1LL

The New Alexander School
21 Lyndhurst Road
Hampstead
London NW3 5NX

North London Alexander School
10 Elmcroft Avenue
London NW11

School of Alexander Studies
44 Park Avenue North
London NW8

Victoria Training Course for the
Alexander Technique
50A Belgrave Road
London SW1

Training

You can apply to be a teacher of the Alexander Technique and you should write to STAT for details. The course lasts three years and costs, on average, £9000. You can train in various parts of the country and STAT will send you a list of approved training courses.

Introductory courses and workshops

Regular half-day introductory courses are held in London. They can take a maximum of five people, cost £24 and last from 10 a.m. to 1 p.m.

Westminster Alexander Centre
8 Hop Gardens
off St Martin's Lane
London WC2N 4EH
Contact: John Hunter

Other Introductory Courses take place around the country. For an up-to-date listing contact STAT, as well as the contacts listed below.

Surrey Contact: James Keating 0181 654 4077
Leicester Contact: Mike Spathaky 01162 715 809
Galway Contact: Immortelle Holistic Centre 0191 61781
Cambridge Contact: Susan Scott-Symons 01223 369 618
Bristol, Bath and Weston-Super-Mare Contact: John Gill
0117 923 7903
York Contact: Jill Freeman 01904 709 688/7684 7917
Windsor Contact: Martin Smith 01753 850 613

Other teaching

For details of Local Authority Adult Education classes in the Alexander Technique, contact your local education authority, the local town hall or your library.

Course are sometimes run abroad. You could try the two listed below for details.

The Skyros Centre
92 Prince of Wales Road
London NW5 3NE

(for holidays, on the Greek island of Skyros, with personal development themes including the Alexander Technique)

Cortijo Romero
c/o Janice Gray
Little Grove
Grove Lane
Chesham
Bucks HP5 3QQ

(alternative holidays in Spain, in the foothills of the Sierra Nevada mountains)

You can always try checking the notice boards of your local health food shops, alternative bookshops and complementary health clinics. They usually have details of any workshops and courses in your area. Otherwise contact STAT.

Bookshops

STAT Books uses its profits to publish material on the Alexander Technique which wouldn't be available otherwise. It is a mail order bookshop although it can be visited during office hours. It has a small selection of 'sold as seen' damaged stock at reduced prices.

STAT Books
20 London House
266 Fulham Road
London SW10 9EL

Books

A wide range of books is available from STAT Books. Some of the books are intended for teachers as teaching aids and aren't really suitable for students as they contain little information of a practical nature. Please check with STAT Books if you are unsure.

All of the books listed in the Bibliography that are specifically on the technique should be available from STAT Books. Some of the others may not be, but you should be able to order them from town centre bookshops or your local library.

Cassettes

Available from STAT Books:

The Alexander Technique by Richard Brennan
The Art of Changing by Glen Park
Body Sense by Sally Tottle

Journals

Available from STAT Books:

The Alexander Journal
The Alexander Review
STAT News
DIRECTION

Videos

Available from STAT Books:

The Alexander Technique: What's That?
Running time 80 minutes. Follows a group of participants in a introductory course to the Technique run by Don Burton at the Fellside Alexander School in 1988.

From Stress to Freedom
Running time 47 minutes. Covers the basic principles.

Posture and Pain
Running time 30 minutes. Produced by the Central Office of Information in 1984 and shown on Channel 4 in the UK.

Chair and cushion accessories

for Balans chairs and wedge cushions, etc:

Pelvic Posture Ltd,
Oaklands
New Mill Lane
Eversley
Hampshire RG27 0RA

You can also try your *Yellow Pages* under 'Medical Supplies'.

BIBLIOGRAPHY

The books included in the Bibliography are recommended. If any are left out, it in no way reflects on them. It just means I haven't read them and therefore cannot recommend them to you as potential sources of information, although I'm quite sure they're fine if STAT Books stock them.

Alexander Technique books

Barker, Sarah, *The Alexander Technique: The Revolutionary Way to Use your body for Total Energy*, Bantam Books, New York, 1978.

Brennan, Richard, *The Alexander Technique: Natural Poise For Health*, Element Books, London, 1991.

Brennan, Richard, *The Alexander Technique Workbook*, Element Books, London, 1992.

Gelb, Michael, *Body Learning: An Introduction to the Alexander Technique*, Aurum Press, London, 1987.

Hodgkinson, Liz, *The Alexander Technique And How It Can Help You*, Piatkus, London, 1988.

Macdonald, Glynn, *The Alexander Technique: Headway Lifeguides*, Hodder & Stoughton, 1994.

Mail, Edward, *The Alexander Technique: The Essential Writings of F. Matthias Alexander*, Thames & Hudson, London, 1974.

Stevens, Chris, *Alternative Health: Alexander Technique*, Optima, London, 1987.

Other useful books

Barlow, Dr Wilfred, *The Alexander Principle*, Victor Gollancz, 1990.

Foulkes, Jane, *Complementary Medicine Careers Handbook*, Hodder & Stoughton, London, 1991.

Hewitt, James *Teach Yourself Relaxation*, Hodder & Stoughton, London, 1992.

Lettvin, Maggie, *The Back Book*, Souvenir Press Ltd, London, 1976.

Mulligan, John, *The Personal Management Handbook: How to Make The Most Of Your Potential*, Sphere Books, London, 1988.

Stanway, Dr Andrew, *Alternative Medicine: A Guide to Natural Therapies*, Bloomsbury Books, London, 1979.

CHAPTER SUMMARY AND CHECKLIST

To save you having to read the whole book each time you want to remind yourself about a particular aspect or principle of the Alexander Technique I include here a quick summary and checklist of each chapter – however don't be tempted to look at these first before you read the whole book. It's important that you not only know the principles but also *why* they apply to learning the Alexander Technique – in a way that's the whole principle – learning conscious choice of what we are doing.

―――――――――― **Chapter 1** ――――――――――

We learnt about Frederick Alexander and how he developed his Technique and why.

Alexander developed his technique out of his own problems of voice loss. He saw the cause as threefold:

- he tensed his neck causing his head to go back
- he tightened his throat muscles
- he took a short deep breath.

He also developed some fundamental principles that can be summed up as:

- the *manner of doing* – how we develop the habits that precede movements
- *not doing* – the more we try to correct the faults the worse we can make it – by not doing we can learn more
- *primary control* – the relationship between head, neck and torso influence the entire body
- *inhibiting* – old habits are stronger that the desire to change – before movement we have a choice whether we begin the movement or not.

Chapter 2

We looked at what the Technique is and learnt some of the important terms associated with the Alexander Technique and what they mean:

- *primary control*
- *conscious projection*
- *end gaining*
- *the means whereby*
- *inhibitions*
- *anti-gravity*
- *function*
- *stimuli*.

Chapter 3

We looked at what the Alexander Technique is for and how it can help. We also looked at some basic principles of:

- responses to stress
- letting go of excess tension
- the *startle pattern*
- the body's defence mechanisms
- internal sensors
- the two types of muscles
- the two systems of muscle nerves
- confusing the system
- the four *stages of doing*
- developing bad habits.

Chapter 4

We looked at who can benefit from learning and applying the Alexander Technique and we decided that anyone can benefit and that once you've learnt it you can:

- apply it to any and all new situations as they occur
- change and adapt it as you change and adapt in your life

- constantly monitor it as you put it into practice
- use it to refresh yourself whenever you feel you're going back to old habits
- find new ways to incorporate it into your daily life.

It's an operating system – once learnt it just sits in the background helping you to operate efficiently.

Chapter 5

We learnt about the Alexander Technique lessons and Alexander Technique teachers and that you should have lessons if you need to correct a particular fault or to check you are using the Technique properly. Some people keep their lessons going on a regular basis for years. Others have one or two and then find they have learnt enough to help them. It's up to you to decide what you need. Have lessons only from a qualified STAT-approved teacher if you feel you want lessons.

Chapter 6

This is the important one – the practical *how to do it for yourself*. We looked at:

- defining the Alexander Technique
- misconceptions about *inhibiting, conscious projecting* and *primary control*
- the best *use* of ourselves
- re-aligning ourselves
- how we get out of alignment
- choosing our seating position
- how our emotions can change our body shape
- a new way of walking
- the *semi-supine*.

Conclusions:

- we need to be constantly adapting and changing
- we need to be aware of how much we move by habit and, if these habits are not done according to the best principles of body design, change them.

Chapter 7

We looked at the practical applications of the Alexander Technique and you learnt how to:

- fill in your chart – be honest and as accurate as you can
- analyse each activity for poor alignment – what could you change? What could you improve? What do you do through habit?
- recognise unconscious signals – see if you're giving any off – they may affect the way people react to you
- think a *head* – your head is important – give it some attention
- try to keep your eyes straight – by starting off straight you end up straight.

Chapter 8

We discussed the human body, how it works and what we do to discourage it from working to the maximum of its efficiency. Remember that the three important principles of allowing the body to operate well, gracefully, efficiently and aligned are:

- *let the neck be free*
- *let the head go forwards and up*
- *allow the back to lengthen and widen.*

Chapter 9

This is where you will find all the useful information such as addresses, details of courses, teachers and workshops.

Remember that there are no rules – there is no right or wrong – there is only allowing the body to perform as it was designed to, or letting it perform badly. Once we know what we are doing to upset our alignment we can choose to continue to do so or we can improve the way we move – it's our choice.

INDEX